First aid for hypochondriacs

First aid for hypochondriacs

by James Gorman

Illustrations by
Henry R. Martin

Workman Publishing
New York

Library of Congress Cataloging in Publication Data

Gorman, James, 1949–
    First aid for hypochondriacs.

        1. Hypochondria—Anecdotes, facetiae, satire, etc.
I. Title
RC552.H8G67   1982   616.85′25′0207   82-60060
ISBN   0-89480-173-2 (pbk.)

Cover design and book: Paul Hanson
Cover illustration: Paul Hanson

Workman Publishing Company, Inc.
1 West 39th Street
New York, N.Y. 10018

Manufactured in the United States of America
First printing September 1982

10 9 8 7 6 5 4 3 2 1

Preface

If you are one of those insufferably good people who like to help old ladies who slip on ice, and who yearn to rush to the aid of avalanche victims, this book isn't for you. Go join a volunteer ambulance society, or give blood to the Red Cross—lots of it.

This book is for people who have enough worries of their own, what with backaches, cancer, and heart disease, people who don't need to participate in mountain rescues to feel that they are gambling with death—swollen glands are risky enough.

These people are hypochondriacs, which means that they—or we, since I count myself among them—care about their health. Never mind all the nonsense about hypochondria being a morbid or excessive concern with the body and health. Is it morbid to worry that a twinge in the chest could be the forerunner of the Big One? Is it excessive to insist that your wife scrub down and sterilize her tweezers before she takes a sliver out of your toe? Is it too much to survey your body daily for the warning signs of cancer? No. No! *No!* Extremism in the defense of health is no vice. Medicine, like charity, begins at home. If you don't look out for your body, no one else will.

Naturally, you will want to have physicians take care of most of your health problems. But in addition to being ridiculously expensive—and often abusive—doctors are seldom available at 2:00 A.M., which is usually when you realize that you are going to die of liver cancer. That's when first aid comes in.

I am deeply indebted for help in preparing this book to the scores of hypochondriacs I know. To protect them, all the facts in the book have been changed. Only the names of the illnesses remain the same. I am also deep in debt to many doctors. However, no physician aided, consulted, or in any way contributed knowledge or information to this book. Everything I know about medicine I taught myself or made up.

J. M. G.

New York, 1982

Contents

5 **Preface**

9 **Introduction**

15 **Sudden illness**

16 **Heart attack**

22 **Stroke**

23 **Allergic reactions**

25 **Appendicitis**

26 **Hiccoughs**

27 **Slower illness**

27 **Brain tumor**

29 **Hemorrhoids**

29 **Cancer**

30 The 10,000 causes of Cancer

31 Warts

33 **Eczema**

34 **Hypoglycemia**

35 **Venereal disease**

36 **Kuru**

37 **Muscle and bone**

37 **The back**

38 Causes of back pain

39 Sex, or the beast with two backs, one aching

40 **Stress fractures**

41 **Twitches and cramps**

43 **Wounds**

43 **Cuts**

45 The ultimate causes of cuts

49 **Contusions**

51 **Dressings with style**

51 **Bandages**

55 **Ace bandages**

56 **Casts**

59 **Shock and disappointment**

59 **Shock**

62 **Disappointment**

65 **Cold comfort**

66 **Colds**

71 **The flu**

72 **Pneumonia**

72 **Bronchitis**

73 How to work a thermometer

74 **Laryngitis**

75 **The breath of life**

76 **Artificial respiration**

76 **Hyperventilation**

77 **Inability to breathe**

79 **Choking**

80 **Sleep apnea**

83 **Poisons**

84 **Food poisoning**

86 **Botulism**

86 **Chemical poisons**

89 **Kitchen surgery**

90 **Slivers**

90 **The med-tech kitchen**

95   **Plague and other horrors**
95   **Plague**
97   **Leprosy**
97   **Rabies**

99   **Travel sickness**
100   Vacations for the ill
103   In hospital abroad
104   Twenty ways to say "I'm sick"
104   **Malaria**
105   **Motion sickness**
106   **Montezuma's revenge**
106   **Parasites**

109   **Out of doors**
110   **The sun**
112   **Hypothermia**
115   **Plants**
116   **Insects**

119   **In the mind**
120   **Depression**
121   **Manic-depressive illness**
122   **Schizophrenia**
123   **Split personality**
124   Free association by hypochondriac
124   Hypochondriac's hypochondriac

125   **The hippocratic curse**
126   **Finding a doctor**
126   **The waiting room**
128   Doctor's horoscope

130   **Doctor-patient etiquette**
132   **The emergency room**
133   Medical diary

Home health care section

137   **Nutrition**
139   **Cholesterol**
139   **Fiber**
140   **Vitamins**
141   A day in the diet
142   **Additives**
142   **The ethics of food**

145   **Exercise**
146   **Muscular fitness**
148   **Aerobic exercise**
151   **Sports**

153   **Medication**
154   **How to read a drug label**
155   **Common and dangerous drugs**
156   How to take a pill
156   **Drug interactions**
157   The hypochondriac's medicine cabinet

159   **How long before you die**

Introduction

A hypochondriac is a person who is concerned about health—ill health, that is. Other people spend a lot of time in foolish worry about how they are going to stay healthy. Should they run marathons? Should they eat grass to stay regular? Hypochondriacs, though they too indulge in foolish worry, know in their hearts that it is impossible to avoid ill health.

If the body doesn't betray you with a sudden failure such as a myocardial infarction, chemicals and radiation are sure to give you cancer. If degenerative arthritis or herpes doesn't afflict you, you are likely to sprain your ankle, or fall prey to lacerations, abrasions, or contusions. The world is full not only of bacteria and poisons, but of sharp objects and hard places to fall. No matter what you do to stay healthy, you are likely to fail.

Hypochondriacs know that the world is an incredibly dangerous place and are surprised—and rightly so—to be alive at all. They expect to be sick. Their only question is: "What is wrong with me today?"

This recognition of the hazards of life and the prevalence of illness fosters a finely tuned attention to all bodily signals, and often causes the hypochondriac to develop a bank of medical knowledge. No disease is too grand, and no symptom too small. In fact, any bodily sensation whatever is suspect. The hypochondriac believes that, like Victorian children, the body should be silent. We all know that we have

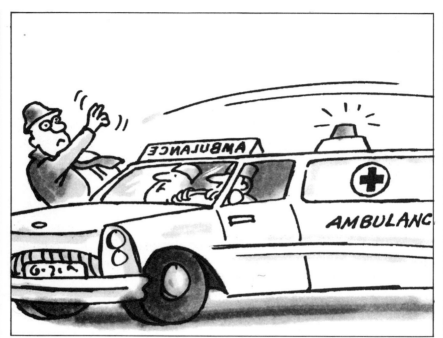

You should know how to hail an ambulance.

knees, but we don't expect to hear from them.

Hypochondriacs suspect emotions as well. Some have been known to mistake an unexpected surge of joy for a killing fever, or a split personality. But hypochondriacs do not make up symptoms. Someone who says he is bleeding when he is not is psychotic, not hypochondriacal. A hypochondriac may, of course, say he is hemorrhaging whenever he sees blood.

Because of their outlook on life, hypochondriacs have many, many medical emergencies, and a heretofore unsatisfied need for their own first aid manual to help them get through these crises.

Most first aid books deal with drowning victims, people who have been mangled in car crashes, and desert hikers who have been bitten by the Sonora sidewinder. This book is different. It does cover snakebite, but only for nonpoisonous species. But it does not tell you how to take care of other people. No hypochondriac has time for other sick people and accident victims. And very few sick people and accident victims have time for hypochondriacs. As a hypochondriac, you are on your own. This book tells you how to take care of yourself when everyone else is sick of you.

First Aid for Hypochondriacs tells you what to do when you see spots in front of your eyes and think you have a brain tumor. It tells you how to perform minor surgery on yourself, thus saving money on medical bills. It tells you how much to tip a doctor, how to find out if you have Elephant Man disease, and what to do if you think you have a split personality. It tells you how to wrap an attractive bandage, how to take your pulse in public, and how to deal with the arrogance of health chauvinists—people who think being sick makes you a sissy.

First Aid for Hypochondriacs is not only about applying gauze pads and Preparation H, but also about learning a certain style, a way of being in the world that will bring you reassurance, support, and perhaps even medical attention from others. Knowing how to sigh can be as impor-tant as learning the Heimlich manuever.

General principles of first aid for hypochondriacs

1. Sickness is like radiation. No level is acceptable. Every illness, every injury from a hangnail to a scratch, is a direct assault on the body and should be taken with the utmost seriousness.

2. The domino theory. The fall of one body part may lead to the fall of others, until the entire mechanism comes toppling down. A head cold can lead to a sore throat; a sore throat to a strep throat. This infection can attack the heart, causing enough damage so that you will later have to undergo open heart surgery. The original cold may spread to the lungs, worsening into pneumonia. The combination of pneumonia and the weakened heart could mean the end. Like communism, sickness must be stopped wherever it starts, with all the resources at your command.

3. Appearance and reality. Nothing is what it seems. A small cut on the finger is not just a small cut. It is a drastic breach in the body's primary defense against the rampant filth and disease of the outside world. Once the skin is broken, disease can enter directly into the body—without having to pass through the nose or the mouth.

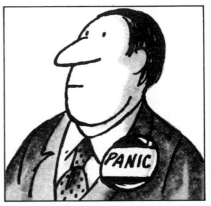

Don't be afraid to panic.

General directions for giving first aid

1. Be prepared. People may laugh at you for having an iron lung in the garage, just in case. But the principle is sound. You never know when you are going to stop breathing.

2. Be bold. "I've got an ulcer" is always a better thing to say than "I think I'm coming down with something."

3. Keep your goals in mind. Do you want immediate medical attention? Or just attention? Do you want a private hospital room, or just a blanket and a cup of tea?

4. Panic. All the advice about not panicking is wishful thinking. When something awful is happening to the body, it knows it and it sends adrenaline and other panic chemicals into the bloodstream. There is no use fighting the body. If you have just stepped on a rusty tack, you and the body both know that you could die from lockjaw. Don't be fooled by the calm words of others who try to hide the truth from you. Let the panic sweep over you in waves. It helps the body fight off bacteria.

If urgent action is required

1. Make sure that you are breathing.

2. Don't bleed.

3. Don't move unless it is necessary (e.g., to get away from a dog or child that has bitten you).

4. Avoid being chilled. Keep a lot of warm sweaters on hand for crises.

5. Determine exactly what has happened. Ask yourself, and anyone else around you, if they remember whether the brand of mushroom soup you had for lunch has been recalled for botulism.

6. Note your general appearance. Do you look yellow? Jaundice always means something, even if you have just fallen down a flight of stairs. Turning blue is a definite danger sign.

7. Are you unconscious?

8. Is your heart beating?

9. Stay in charge until the doctor arrives. If you let someone else take over, they are likely to tell you to have a drink or go to sleep. They may even call the doctor and tell him not to come at all.

10. Be sure to have your own diagnosis and treatment plan ready when the doctor arrives.

Sudden illness

The frightening thing about the body is that it is subject to failure at any moment. This is particularly true of the heart. Of course, the brain and the feet are also subject to sudden attack, but in most people these are not vital organs. The heart is.

The problem for the hypochondriac is how to face life with a treacherous and unreliable body. Once you have taken your pulse and felt the pathetic little thumping on which your life depends, how can the thought of heart failure ever be out of your mind? The answer is that it can't; and moreover, it shouldn't be.

As a hypochondriac you should always expect sudden illness to strike. Even so, like a Londoner during the Blitz, you will still be taken by surprise when the raid on your heart does come. All you can do is try to be vigilant. Like the English people at war, who never ignored a siren, you should never ignore a symptom. You are at war with illness. You must fight it in the pharmacies, you must fight it in the emergency rooms, you must fight it in the sickroom. You must stop it—with toil, tears, and sweat. Not blood; if you have to bleed, you've already lost.

The way to exercise vigilance is to take your pulse. Of course, this gives you no clues about appendicitis or stroke. And it is exceedingly difficult to monitor the appendix or the brain. The former does nothing and the latter has its finger (so to speak) in everything. At any rate, you are far more liable to get a heart at-

Heart attack

tack than anything else. Stick to your pulse.

When sudden illness does strike—or seem to strike—first aid usually consists of trying to calm yourself down. This may involve the sort of activity that makes other people extremely excited, particularly if you are in public. The key to carrying off the actions that first aid may require is never to apologize. If your suspicion that you are dying has convinced your favorite co-worker to give you mouth-to-mouth resuscitation in the building lobby, and it turns out that your pains were the result of gas, do not act embarrassed. This will only make your co-worker feel bad. She will start asking herself why she was on her knees breathing in your mouth in front of all those people. Just tell her that she saved your life, and impress her with how grateful you are.

Heart attack

There are many kinds of heart attacks. Doctors tend to focus on the ones where the heart actually stops beating, or where a coronary artery shuts down like the Long Island Expressway at rush hour. This is a typical physician's point of view, far too limited for hypochondriacs, who have heart attacks all the time. In fact, there are as many kinds of heart attacks as there are hypochondriacs. The ones you should worry about the most are: the Big One and the Different Drummer.

The big one

This is it, the ultimate bodily betrayal, a massive myocardial infarction. A blocked coronary artery shuts off blood to the heart, part or all of which dies.

Ninety-nine out of a hundred times when you think the Big One has finally gotten you, you will be wrong. Never mind. The whole point about precipitous and deadly illnesses such as heart attacks is that they are so bad you can't afford to ignore them, even if you aren't having them. Pay close attention to the faintest symptoms.

The Big One can strike anywhere, at any time—at home, on the bus, or at a dinner party. The symptoms are always the same.

☞   **Signs and symptoms**

1. A large pain taking up most of your chest and

Heart attack

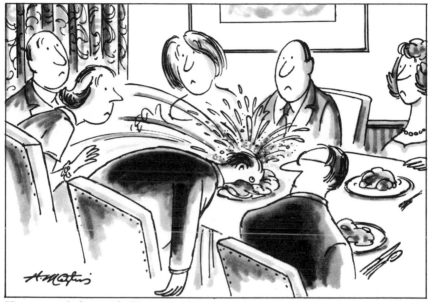

Heart attack first aid: First, get their attention.

sometimes stretching down your arm. The size of the pain is as important as its intensity. The greater the surface area it covers, the worse the heart attack. Weight is also important. Heart attack pains are very heavy. A bad attack will feel as if a doctor's golf bag has been dropped on your chest.

2. Fatty visions. Hypochondriacs have a sixth sense for cholesterol, and often see it in their mind's eye clogging and cluttering their arteries. These visions are particularly strong during suspected heart attacks.

3. Fear. It is as significant as pain. Sometimes the pain will be faint, but the fear massive. Treat this as a major heart attack. Fear evolved as a protective device over millions of years. Why would you be afraid if nothing were happening to you?

4. A sense of doom. This feeling is known to accom-

Heart attack

pany very bad heart attacks. If you sense that you will never see your cardiologist again, go to him immediately.

✚ First aid

Actual medical care for the Big One involves oxygen tents and cardiac emergency teams and cardiologists. What you can do for yourself is make sure that the fear that you are about to die doesn't kill you. In extreme cases you can pick up the telephone and call your local ambulance service. They can, however, be very nasty if it turns out that you had indigestion. For self-help, you can take some less drastic measures first. What you do depends on whether you are alone or with others.

In private

1. Take your pulse. Always take your pulse. The heart has to know that you are in charge. If it is thinking of quitting, a good firm finger on the pulse may scare it into staying on the job. You can feel your pulse either at your wrist or at the carotid artery in your neck, just behind the windpipe.

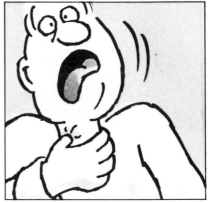

Taking your pulse, obtrusively.

Or, with a little practice, you can tune in to your body so that you can just listen to the blood flowing through your ears. This is particularly effective when you are lying with your ear pressed against a pillow.

2. Get somebody quick. Try to get them to give you CPR.* If they won't, then ask them if you look like you are having a heart attack.

3. Call your heart's bluff.

*Cardiopulmonary resuscitation—heart massage and mouth-to-mouth resuscitation. Try to get family members to take courses in CPR so they will be prepared.

Heart attack

If nobody is around and you are left with the choice of calling the ambulance or taking care of yourself, there is one sure way to determine whether you are having a heart attack: Pick a long flight of stairs and run up it as fast as you can. This will often relieve gas pains, but it has the opposite effect on heart attacks. Be sure to have a telephone at the top of the stairs (or better, halfway up) in case you want to call the ambulance when you get there.

In public

The Big One more often occurs at dinner parties where something like Boeuf Mort de la Beurre (beef drowned in butter) is being served. The situation is particularly frightening because people at dinner parties do not like other people to have heart attacks during the meal. They will ignore all but the most obvious signs of illness in favor of keeping the conversation going.

When the attack begins:

1. Take your pulse. You can do this unobtrusively or obtrusively.

(a) UNOBTRUSIVELY. Put your hands under the table, or casually rest your chin in your hand, letting your thumb slide down to the carotid artery in your neck.

(b) OBTRUSIVELY. You may want other people to see you, in hopes that they will spring to your aid.

Hold your left wrist up as if you were about to shake your fist and then place the first three fingers of the right hand on the artery. Someone may interpret this as an obscene gesture, or they may ask you what you think of Steven Spielberg. This means you have failed to get their attention.

Or ask someone else to take your pulse. But be aware that few people know your pulse as well as you do. At most, they will be able to tell you whether your heart is beating. And you can't always trust them even for that; it may be their own pulse they are feeling. Remember: A man

Heart attack

who lets a stranger take his pulse has a fool for a doctor.

2. If your heart is beating, only reassurance is needed. Try to turn the talk around to your symptoms to see if anyone else is having them (or thinks they sound bad). A good way to start such a conversation is to ask around the table whether anyone has had an electrocardiogram recently.

3. If your heart is not beating, you must try to galvanize the dinner party to come to your aid and get you to a hospital where you can get professionals to take your pulse. Don't forget that your companions know you, and know you are a hypochondriac.

(a) Don't say, "I'm having a heart attack." Most people feel that if a known hypochondriac is healthy enough to make intelligible sounds there is nothing wrong with him.

(b) Do fall face forward into your plate. Nobody would believe that you would do this if you

weren't really sick.

(c) Don't turn blue or act like you are having trouble breathing. If you do, someone might think that you are choking and punch you in the stomach.

The different drummer

This is a different sort of heart attack, in which the heart goes off its beat. It happens to people with unreliable hearts that are always losing track of their rhythm. It is not so much a blatant betrayal as it is cardiac negligence.

The Big One comes only once in a lifetime, but if you have a forgetful heart, you will experience these small attacks all the time. This is no reason to take them lightly. They could always signal the start of fibrillation, in which the heart loses all regularity and starts quivering uselessly. Death follows swiftly.

☞ **Signs and symptoms**

1. Suddenly you feel a little *bub-a-loop* in your chest and you know that your heart is having what doctors call a cardiac arrythmia, or, in English, a heart

Heart attack

with no rhythm. In reality, the heart may just not have the rhythm you want it to have. But the body is not a democracy, and if you feel as though Gene Kelly is tap dancing on the inside of your ribs, you must set the heart straight.

✚ First aid

1. Once again, take your pulse. If you are subject to these attacks, and many hypochondriacs get them several times a day, you should take it regularly, every fifteen minutes or so, just in case.

2. Put pressure on the heart. Try bringing it back to its senses by squeezing your chest together. This can also slow down a heart that starts beating too fast. This is called tachycardia (or, tacky heart).

3. Try homeopathic medicine and start dancing yourself. This often quiets the heart. (Sometimes it silences it completely, but all treatments have their risks.) Dancing works because it is a message to the heart to

stop fooling around and start pumping blood to the legs and feet.

⇒ Prevention

Aside from taking your pulse there are some other things that you can do to aid your heart and keep it beating well. The legs are sometimes called "the second heart" because their muscular action helps pump blood throughout the body. You can aid in this action when you are standing still.

1. Rise up on the balls of your feet frequently to keep the muscles active. In company, you can do this imperceptibly so that, at worst, the people around you think that you are of a nervous nature.

2. Exercise "the third heart"—the arms. While sitting, at a play, for instance, clench and unclench your fists to aid the heart. Take a break every once in a while to check on your pulse. If you are going out with someone for the first time, it is best to

Stroke

explain your actions beforehand, since this sort of
behavior can be distracting
to others.

Stroke

As everyone knows, different
folks have different strokes. Some
leave the victim completely para-
lyzed. Others only paralyze parts
of the body. All paralyzing
strokes, however, are major
strokes, far beyond the capabili-
ties of first aid.

But as a hypochondriac you
also have to worry about minor
strokes, which are only noticeable
because of a slight dizziness and
loss of memory. A small part of
the brain is lost, and some thinking power may go with it. If you
weren't keeping track of everything going on in your body, you
might never notice one of these
strokes.

These sudden illnesses can
be treated with first aid, and often
leave no lasting effects, which is
where the phrase "a stroke of
good luck" comes from.

☞ **Signs and symptoms**

1. Spots before your eyes.
Medical science has not
determined whether spots
in front of the eyes are the
result of a brain tumor, a
stroke, incipient blindness,
or pushing on your eye-
balls with your fingers. As
a hypochondriac you have
to be wary of anything un-
usual. Assume the worst.

2. Sleeping limbs. You
wake up at night and you
can't move your arm. It is
cold and has no feeling.
You may suspect that
someone has put a dead
salmon in your bed. The
common explanation for
this experience is that the
arm has fallen asleep, but
it is always possible that it
has been knocked out cold
by a clot in the brain. Slap
it and massage it to wake it
up. If it doesn't come to,
see a doctor.

3. Confusion and forgetful-
ness. The most common
symptoms of small strokes.
Remember this when you
are accused by your spouse
of forgetting to take a roll
of film to be developed for
the twelfth day in a row.
Say, "I can't believe I for-
got that. I must have had a
small stroke."

Allergic reactions

✚ First aid

1. Give the brain some rest. Stop playing chess; don't read Henry James. (This also works for head colds.)

2. Go on a no-salt diet. Salt contributes to atherosclerosis, which is a cause of heart attacks and stroke. Try to convince your entire family that because of genetic susceptibility, what could happen to you could happen to them. Hide the salt shakers.

3. Use a cane and complain of generalized muscle weakness. You won't be lying. There are no strong hypochondriacs. Be sure to get a cane with a crook handle and a rubber tip; otherwise it will look like a walking stick and observers may think you are a dandy rather than someone who is seriously ill.

Allergic reactions

What you have to worry about with allergies is not the sneezing and the wheezing, or the hives and nausea. Of course, you will want to call everyone's attention to these symptoms, but the real problem is anaphylactic shock— an allergic reaction so severe that it can kill you.

Anything that can cause allergies can cause anaphylactic shock—plums, eggplant, cats, horses, penicillin, or other people. Many people who don't have any obvious allergies do not worry about anaphylactic shock. But you should realize that there are many things that you have never been exposed to. You don't know whether you are allergic to them. This means that any new food, animal, medicine, or person could kill you. This possibility makes it hard for a hypochondriac to be adventurous in life.

☛ Signs and symptoms

1. Breathlessness. This is always a symptom of something, if only lack of oxygen. If you have just been exposed to something you don't like, it might be the beginning of anaphylaxis.

2. Sneezing. Does not usually lead to death, but could signal a new allergy,

Allergic reactions

which might become more dangerous on the second exposure.

3. Pallor. A sudden lack of color on exposure to something you are allergic to. The appearance of liver and onions on your plate may do this to you. If this happens, don't eat them. Plead a serious allergy.

4. Collapse. Often occurs with allergies to large pets, such as Great Danes. Sometimes collapse is merely the result of the pet leaping on you, but this does not mean you aren't allergic to it.

✚ First aid

The basic principle of first aid for allergies is to get away from the bad thing. Sometimes this can be done by simply saying, "I'm allergic to animals, if you make me hold your mouse I might throw up." Sometimes more extreme measures are called for.

Food allergies

If it's already on your plate and they are trying to make you eat it:

1. Taste the offending item.

2. Say, "Oh, my God, is that eggplant?" and spit it out on the plate.

3. You have now made all the other people at the table so disgusted that they are speechless. Apologize, and explain that you are allergic to eggplant. You can be confident no one will ever serve it to you again. In fact, no one is likely to speak to you again. This is the price of illness.

Pet allergies

Many pet owners don't believe in allergies. They suspect that people who claim to be allergic to dogs, for example, just don't like to have their faces licked by creatures whose idea of fun is to roll in dead fish. Dog owners consider this to be inexcusable effeteness. To impress them with the reality of your allergy, as soon as you see the animal, screech in high, panicky tones, "I'm allergic to dogs! I'm allergic to dogs! I'm allergic to dogs!" It is necessary to say it at least

Appendicitis

three times, because the first time dog owners won't hear you, and the second time they won't believe you. The same procedure should be followed for cats, gerbils, and boa constrictors.

Appendicitis

All hypochondriacs have an attack of apparent appendicitis at some point in their careers. Many of them have appendicitis regularly. It always comes on suddenly, and always at an inconvenient time.

☞ Signs and symptoms

1. A pain in the side. This always occurs while you are alone, or with someone who doesn't know which side your appendix is on.

2. You are never sure which side your appendix is on.

✚ First aid

1. The first thing to do is to find out which side your appendix is on. Nothing is more embarrassing than going to the emergency room with appendicitis only to find that your pain is on the wrong side. Any medical book can tell you where your appendix is.

2. Determine whether you have had your appendix removed. If your memory is fuzzy, remember that they give you ice cream after a tonsillectomy, not an appendectomy. If you just don't know, call your mother. She'll probably be happy to hear from you anyway. If she doesn't know, and if you have no abdominal scars, you probably have your appendix.

3. If the pain stops, this means either that your appendix has burst and you are going to die, or that you never had appendicitis to start with and you simply shouldn't eat onions for lunch. To be safe, you should go to the emergency room and explain that though you feel fine at the moment, a little while before you were in pain. Whether or not you want to take this course of action depends on which you fear more, embarrassment or death.

Hiccoughs

Hiccoughs

Most hypochondriacs know that people have died of hiccoughs. Unable to stop hiccoughing, their humorous spasms ended in death. If you are aware of this possibility, the laughter of your friends while you hiccough may only increase your fear.

Imagine, in your twentieth day of hiccoughing, as you approach the end, each *hic* is so feeble the *up* is almost lost. Your so-called friends are laughing so hard that they are weeping and cannot see through their tears that you are on your way out. It is a classic hypochondriac's fate, to die while a crowd of people looks on laughing in disbelief.

Treat hiccoughs seriously. Take these quick first aid steps.

✚ First aid

1. Inform the people around you that hiccoughs are actually respiratory spasms, which are not funny.

2. Swallow sugar, or drink a glass of water backwards. (To do this, simply drink the water from the side of the glass farthest away from your mouth. If this sounds too complicated, try the sugar.)

3. Keep saying to everyone, "It's not—*(hic)*—funny."

4. Finally, point out that people have also died from laughing.

Case history

A woman at work received a puzzling call from her husband (a cardiac hypochondriac), who seldom telephoned her during the day unless he felt ill. This time he seemed strangely silent about his health.

"Well," she said, "how are you?"

"Better than Harold," he replied.

"What happened to Harold?" she asked. Harold was a friend of her husband's and about the same age. Both men were in their early forties.

"He had a heart attack. That's what happened to him."

The woman was stunned, and said how awful the news was.

"Yes," replied the man with a tone of righteousness. "So let's hear no more about hypochondria."

Slower illness

Tomorrow, and tomorrow, and tomorrow, creeps in this petty pace. And so do most illnesses. But although the illness may be slow, the realization that you've got it usually strikes with the speed of a heart attack. There is a moment when every hypochondriac realizes that he has been eating hot dogs for years, that hot dogs cause cancer, and that by inescapable logic, he must have cancer. You can't go to the emergency room with a problem like that; you can't even go to a doctor. You need first aid.

Furthermore, you will find that no matter how slow the illness, the doctor who treats it is slower. Take eczema. It is very, very slow. But compared to dermatologists, eczema moves at the speed of light. Taking advantage of the stately progression of the diseases they treat, dermatologists are always booked up many weeks in advance, and always make you wait at least 45 minutes in the waiting room (this is a rule of the American Dermatological Association).

Of course, some slow illnesses can be cared for at home, without recourse to doctors. For many of these illnesses, however, doctors are necessary. And it is in the interim between the onset of the disease and the arrival of your doctor's appointment that first aid is necessary for survival.

Brain tumor

The degree of control over the body exercised by the brain

Brain tumor

makes all hypochondriacs nervous. Most of the brain, particularly the part that runs the body, is not conscious. You never know what it is up to or what is happening to it. So you have to be constantly on the lookout for signs of danger.

Because of the scope of the brain's responsibilities, these signs are readily available. The brain affects vision, speech, walking, the emotions, thinking, and most of the body's other functions. Therefore, almost *anything* is a symptom of a brain tumor.

These tumors are the main preoccupation of intellectual hypochondriacs. Beautiful women fear that their skin will rot. Smart people fear that their brains will rot. Smart people who are also beautiful have to worry about everything.

☞ Signs and symptoms

1. Headaches. They should always be treated as symptoms of a tumor.

2. Odd tastes and smells. If you suddenly taste shrimp scampi in the middle of a tennis game, either you had shrimp scampi for lunch or you have a brain tumor. In either case you should stop the game.

3. Spots in front of your eyes. This could also be a stroke. (*See* Stroke.)

4. Odd emotions. Don't worry about depression or sadness, there are always legitimate reasons to feel bad. But be suspicious of so-called "good" emotions, such as giddiness or elation. There is seldom anything in external reality that causes these feelings. They are almost invariably the result of mental illness or a neurological disorder.

✚ First aid

1. Check your sensations and emotions with others around you. Ask them whether they smell onions, taste chalk, or feel unaccountably happy.

2. Do these quick home neurological tests:
(a) Scratch the bottom of your foot. If it makes your ears wiggle, see a neurologist.
(b) Cross your legs and hit your knee with a hammer. Your leg should jerk forward. If you experience in-

Hemorrhoids

tense pain, you are using the wrong kind of hammer.

3. Get a CAT scan. This is a whole-brain X-ray, one of the most exciting new medical procedures available to hypochondriacs. Be sure to keep a copy of the results for your files.

Hemorrhoids

The hidden sorrow. Hemorrhoids are one of the few ailments that not even a hypochondriac wants to talk about.

☞ Signs and symptoms

1. Difficulty sitting still.
2. Difficulty sitting.

✚ First aid

1. Don't ride a bicycle with a racing seat.

2. Soothing creams and treatments offer only temporary relief. For a cure, you need to cauterize the hemorrhoids with fiery foods.

(a) The favored medication is hot sauce. Put hot sauce on everything you eat— scrambled eggs, filet of sole, artichokes, asparagus

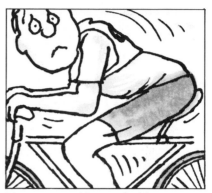

The sorrow of hemorrhoids.

with hollandaise, Boston cream pie.

(b) If you don't like hot sauce because it seems gastronomically tacky, try "haute" hot cuisine— Szechuan food and Indian dishes. The result will be the same and they won't cancel your subscription to *Gourmet.*

Cancer

Cancer may well be the hypochondriac's most common preoccupation. If you are not worried about having it, you are not a hypochondriac.

The most significant thing about cancer, from the hypochondriac's point of view, is its slowness. It can be building in your

Cancer

The 10,000 causes of cancer (partial listing)

the sun
sadness
bacon
too much sleep
too little sleep
the Pill
cigarettes
water
meat
coffee
tea
too little sex
too much sex
the wrong kind of sex
saccharin
hormones
peanut butter
air pollution
hot foods
snuff
color television
X-rays
nuclear power
nuclear war
the nuclear family
asbestos
pesticides
crowding
loneliness
disco music
PCBs
PBBs
DBCP
LSD
STP
STD
Agent Orange
Red Dye #2
glue
varnish
viruses
paint
science
the government
doctors
them

body—starting from a small error in the DNA in one of your cells—for years before it actually erupts in one of the danger signs. Therefore, lack of symptoms means absolutely nothing. You can feel perfectly fine and still not be healthy. This means that a doctor can never say for sure that you don't have cancer.

☞ Signs and symptoms

1. Moles. Moles are the early warning system of

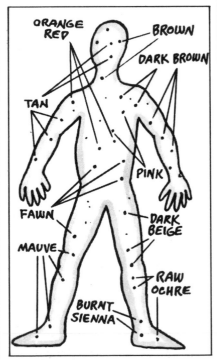

Sample mole map.

Cancer

Warts

Your first thought when you find an ugly growth on your skin will naturally be that you have cancer. Not so fast. If it is really ugly, it is probably a wart. And warts are usually not signs of cancer, even though they look like they should be.

Having warts is not the kind of medical problem you want to get involved in, primarily because of their ugliness. There is a lot of sympathy and attention to be had for being sick. But being ugly gets you nowhere.

However, there is really no way to avoid getting warts. According to doctors, warts are caused by viruses, not toads. Of course, this is no reason to assume that toads don't carry the viruses that cause warts. And even if toads are perfectly safe,

there is nothing to be lost by not touching them.

Some warts are frozen off by doctors, others can be chased away at home by the application of castor oil, externally. But new research offers another idea: Warts, perhaps because they are so unattractive, are psychologically sensitive. Hypnotized people have been told that warts will disappear from one side of their body only, and the suggestion has worked.

To try the same thing at home, ignore the warts; pretend they are not there. Don't look at them; don't take them to the doctor; don't put makeup on them. Soon, being sensitive to the psychological currents in the host body, the warts themselves will come to think they are not there and they will fade away.

cancer detection. If a new one appears, or an old one starts to grow, this is a sign of cancer. Draw a map of all the moles on your body, complete with their colors and sizes. With this chart, you will be able to pick out any change immediately. Examine your

moles frequently—not as often as you take your pulse, but more often than you see your psychiatrist.

2. Unexplained itching. A little-known cancer warning. An itching mole is double trouble.

3. Inappropriate bleeding.

Cancer

Moles are not supposed to bleed. If they do, watch out. If they are bleeding, itching, and growing, you don't have much time left.

4. Hair. Losing a lot of it is bad. Gaining a lot of it, in unexpected places, is worse.

✚ First aid

1. Complain. It is well known that anxiety, stress, and tension cause cancer. For hypochondriacs this raises the truly awful possibility that worrying about cancer can cause it. This is, of course, yet another thing to worry about. Although this seems like an endless circle of anxiety, there is a way to break it. Constant moaning and whining is a great reliever of tension. It may give other people cancer, but you will feel much better.

2. Diet. Eat only collard greens and kohlrabi. This may not work, but you will feel that you are taking medicine, and that will make you feel better.

3. Resignation. Being a whiner is not the only way to deal with the certainty that you are dying of a horrible illness while no one believes you. Another alternative is being a saint. Adopt a pose of long-suffering stoicism and great courage. Don't ever mention your disease by name, or use words to describe how you feel. Silences can speak volumes, particularly if they are accompanied by horrible faces.

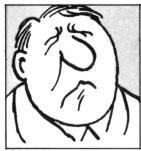

Courage.

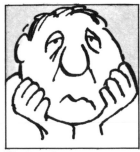

Resignation.

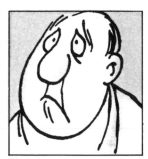

Stoicism.

Eczema

Case history

A young man who was an exceptionally good student in high school was admitted to Harvard. Despite his excellent record and test scores, he found it hard to believe that he had gotten into the most prestigious school in the country.

He began to think that there was only one explanation: He had leukemia. His doctor, family, and school officials all knew. None of them would tell him, but they had told Harvard. And they had made a special plea that he be admitted to make the last few years of his life more satisfying.

He survived Harvard, and graduate school, and is now quite successful, although still concerned about his health. He has concluded that either the leukemia is chronic and very low-level, or he had a spontaneous remission. Which doesn't mean that it won't re-appear.

Eczema

Eczema is what pays for the Mercedes that dermatologists

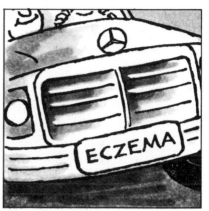

The wages of skin.

drive. Otherwise, there is some disagreement on precisely what the term eczema means. Basically it is a kind of corrosion. What rust does to a Mercedes, eczema does to the skin. It can be caused by anything from worry to having water touch your skin. Eczema should not be confused with some other common skin ailments.*

☞ Signs and symptoms

1. Dryness and flaking on the scalp. This is probably dandruff, a disease in its own right.

2. Big flakes of skin coming off all over the body, accompanied by intense itching. This is called peel-

*If you not only have terrible skin, but your body starts to go all out of shape as well, see a doctor immediately. You could have Elephant Man disease.

Hypoglycemia

ing. It is the result of a sunburn, and you should know better. If you haven't been in the sun recently, see a doctor immediately, or a veterinarian—you have mange.

3. Skin is like sandstone—dry, red and cracking—except for the oozing. This is eczema.

✚ First aid

1. Relax. Laid-back people never have eczema.

2. Go into analysis to find out the underlying cause of the nervousness. Do you hate your mother? Are you allergic to cats? Do you hate cats? Are you allergic to your mother?

3. Protect your body from soap, water, and air.

Hypoglycemia

It is almost impossible to know if you have hypoglycemia, low blood sugar, since its symptoms are so common in anyone who suffers from hypochondria. Once a coveted disease, it has become déclassé because of its popularity among film stars.

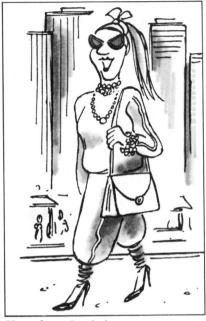

Hypoglycemia victim.

☞ Signs and symptoms

1. Anxiety, sweating, and excitement. These symptoms may also accompany sex, so check to see if you are alone.

2. Delirium and coma. May also be the result of intense interpersonal relations.

3. The above symptoms are ambiguous, but if you have them and you (a) live in California, or (b) wear de-

Venereal disease

signer sweat pants, you probably do have hypoglycemia. At the least you will find a doctor who says you do.

✚ First aid

Change your diet.

1. Stop eating those foods that have lots of sugar so you won't experience a big drop in blood sugar shortly after eating.

2. Eat candy bars and peanut brittle nonstop. This will give you hyperglycemia, high blood sugar, a newer and better syndrome.

Venereal disease

Doctors are now calling VD by a new acronym—STD (for Sexually Transmitted Diseases). This new name is not expected to last long since people are now constantly confusing syphilis with motor oil. Doctors are getting sick of answering victims who ask, "So why do they call it 'the racer's edge'?"

At puberty, all hypochondriacs become terrified of VD, and they have never believed the ru-

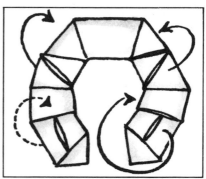

Origami toilet seat cover.

mor that you can't catch it from toilet seats. All hypochondriacs make little paper seat covers whenever they are in a strange bathroom. Not only does it prevent disease, but, like the Japanese art of origami (paper folding), it calms the mind.

Recently, medical science caught up with hypochondria when some scientists reported that although syphilis and gonorrhea do require sexual contact, the new scourge of the sexual revolution—herpes virus—can live for up to 72 hours outside of the body on, for example, toilet seats, or doorknobs. Just as you always suspected, you don't have to have sex to have VD.

Doctors make a number of distinctions between one venereal disease and another, but all share certain characteristics.

Kuru

☞ Signs and symptoms

1. Pimples in unexpected places.

2. Rashes, anywhere.

3. Strange thoughts. Mental illness is one of the signs of the latter stages of syphilis. Hypochondriacs are always afraid that they might have missed the early stages, and are going insane without knowing it, all because of the time they didn't cover the toilet seat in that gas station on Route 72.

✘ Causes

1. The sexual revolution. The idea that it is okay to have sex with more than one person during your lifetime is the main cause of VD.

2. Singles bars. If you go to one, don't use the bathroom.

3. Sexual contact with strangers. (Sexual contact is anything more than a cool "hello.")

✚ First aid

Get VD tests every time you have a checkup, even if you haven't slept with anybody in the past year.

⇒ Prevention

1. Never use a bathroom outside of your home.

2. Sleep only with people who belong to your church.

3. Don't touch doorknobs in public places. Who knows who used them?

Kuru

Kuru is caused by a member of a small and very exclusive group of pathogens called "slow" viruses. They sneak into the body, causing no disturbance when they enter, and then several years later they strike.

Kuru, which is fatal, affects the brain. It was discovered in the mountains of New Guinea, among people who caught it by eating the brains of their deceased relatives. It has been found only in these tribes in New Guinea. So far.

☞ Signs and symptoms

Same as for brain tumor.

✚ First aid

First aid for kuru consists only of prevention.
Never eat brains, whether or not they belong to your relatives.

Muscle and bone

It is apparent to anyone who has spent any time walking around in the human body that it was not well designed. Muscles and bones do not stand up well under the pull of gravity and the force of movement. Not only is the body not well designed for walking (let alone running), it seems to be poorly set up for lifting, pulling, and pushing, and is not all that good for sitting. Even prolonged periods of lying down can cause aches and pains.

The big design flaw in the body is the musculoskeletal system. This consists of the back, neck, knees, and ankles. The musculoskeletal system is ministered to by physicians called orthopedic surgeons. The fact that they are surgeons should tell you something about the musculoskel-etal system. It is the home of the slipped disc, the bone chip, water on the knee, arthritis, and the muscle cramp, as well as the majority of indiscriminate aches and pains that you experience during the day. If you exercise, you can eliminate some of these pains. However, you are likely to cause others. (*See* Exercise.)

Fortunately, first aid for musculoskeletal ailments is often quite pleasant. It usually consists of hot baths and extended periods of total inactivity. It is necessary to have a supportive family, or servants, to practice these techniques correctly.

The back

The back is the major location of pain in the body. Other parts of

The back

the body may send quick telegraphic flashes of pain to the brain, but the back writes long baroque letters.

Because of its tendency to produce pain, the back is all but useless for any physical activity. For this reason, you should avoid lifting anything that requires more than one hand and try to stay away from sports that require a lot of movement.

Causes of back pain

Standing	Stretching
Sitting	Grabbing
Lying down	Carrying
Bending	Pushing
Reaching	Pulling
Lifting	Tugging
Turning	Jerking
Lurching	Toting
Twisting	Hauling
Walking	Squatting
Jumping	Leaning
Skipping	Kneeling
Jogging	Crawling
Hopping	Climbing
Tripping	Clambering
Twirling	Slipping
Whirling	Falling
Leaping	

The back does, however, have its uses. Like the coal miner's canary, it is an early warning system for physical and psychological stress. If you feel a pain in your back, you know you, or somebody, is doing something wrong. If your boss is planning your transfer to a small town in a cold climate, this can cause terrific pains in the upper back and shoulders. If an efficiency expert is about to visit your department, the lower back may tie itself into a knot, making it impossible to sit at a desk. You find you have to lie down at home for several days, or until the crisis is past. You explain to your boss that people in pain do not work efficiently.

☞ **Signs and symptoms**

1. Lower back pain—nagging. Usually the result of a bad chair or boss.

2. Lower back pain—intense. You are unable to bend, or move at all, without pain. Either you have slipped a disc or you are about to be fired. Or both.

3. Middle back pain. Sharp, stabbing sensations when you move the wrong way. (Sometimes all ways

The back

Sex, or the beast with two backs, one aching

People who get romantically involved with hypochondriacs must be willing to accept a lot of infirmities, but they often draw the line at lovemaking. However, if you have a bad back, sex can be dangerous. A strong back for both parties is essential to most forms of sexual intercourse. (This is why lovemaking is called the beast with two backs—one is not enough.) If your back is aching, particularly if it is threatening to slip a disc (lower back pain, moving rapidly from nagging to intense), you probably should not engage in any sexual activity in which you have to move. It could leave you permanently crippled.

pain. This can put your head in a permanently tilted position. Caused by domestic tension or sleeping by an open window. Try eliminating all breezes before you see a marriage counselor.

✚ First aid

1. Walk bent over. Many sufferers of back pain find this technique to be of some relief. You can walk bent over forward or to one side. You can't walk bent over backward. Walking bent over won't cure you,

of moving are wrong.) This is a muscle injury and it is usually the result of unnecessarily vigorous physical activity, such as grocery shopping.

4. Upper back and neck

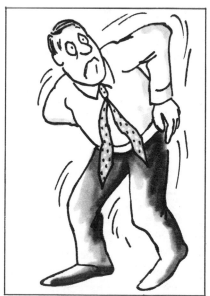

For back pain, walk bent over.

Stress fractures

but it will relieve the pain and it makes people sympathetic in a way that constant complaining could never do.

2. Lie down. This is the best treatment for all sorts of back pain. Do not do anything that requires you to stand, sit, or put any stress on the back. This includes cooking, dishwashing, typing, and having dinner with people you don't like. (True friends will let you eat on the couch.)

3. Moderate exercise. Be careful, because if your pain is caused by a slipped disc, the wrong movements could land you in the hospital. Bend over and touch your upper thighs. Take deep breaths. Walk around the living room.

Stress fractures

Obviously, the bones in the musculoskeletal system can get broken. You will no doubt have the good sense not to put yourself in situations where broken bones are a common occurrence—violent sports, rock climbing, country-and-western bars.

But there is more than one way to break a bone, and the one that you should watch out for particularly is the stress fracture. Of course, this is more common in Thoroughbred horses and marathon runners than it is in hypochondriacs. (Anyone who manages to run a marathon is by definition not a hypochondriac.) You can put a lot of stress on a tibia running 12 miles a day on asphalt. But the stress of walking down Madison Avenue on a crowded afternoon, or trying not to squirm in a tense business meeting, cannot be underestimated. We are all subject to stress, not only physical, but psychological.

● **Types of stress fractures**

1. Stroller's surprise. Excessive walking can result in violent injury, particularly where there are curbs. One misstep, and the strain on a bone can be too much.

2. Pressure break. This is similar to a tension headache. The difference is that the muscles tense up in the

Twitches and cramps

shin or the arm, causing a fracture. This may happen in a bad business meeting or at a family reunion.

☞ Signs and symptoms

1. A broken bone, even if it is only a small fracture, causes intense pain.

2. If it is a leg bone, difficulty walking.

3. If it is an arm bone, difficulty hailing an ambulance.

✚ First aid

1. Get an X-ray. Keep a copy for your files. You may want to check it over to see if the doctor missed anything. If he argues, point out that you paid for the film and the developing.

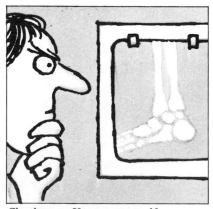

Check your X-rays yourself.

2. Demand a cast. (*See* Dressings with Style.)

3. Avoid physical and emotional stress.

Twitches and cramps

The musculoskeletal system also includes muscles, which have their own peculiarities, primary among them being twitches and cramps. These are apparently unguided actions of the muscles. Nothing is more frightening to the hypochondriac than when parts of the body normally under conscious control, such as the muscles, start acting on their own.

The muscles are not supposed to be independent, for obvious reasons. You don't want your body running off to the supermarket when you have sleeping to do. You don't want to find yourself dancing to disco music, ever. This is why the mind is given dominion over the muscles, most of the time.

At times, however, the body rebels. Tired of kowtowing to the mind, and following instructions such as "Eat that third éclair" or "Watch the late movie," the body decides to take control and

Twitches and cramps

do something on its own. Fortunately, the body is not used to the exercise of power. When it tries for a run in the park, the only result is a throbbing leg muscle or a painful spasm—in other words, a twitch or a cramp. These illnesses come on very suddenly and can always be taken as a sign that the body feels abused.

☞ Signs and symptoms

1. The dying foot. This usually happens at night, as you are turning over in bed. Suddenly the foot curls up as if it belonged to a girl from ancient China, and a searing pain strikes the instep. If this ever occurs in the calf or thigh, it can cripple you for life.
2. The twitch. This can happen anywhere on the body and consists of a muscle that should not be working at all trembling and throbbing. The twitch can be frightening, since it looks as if there were a small lizard undergoing a painful death just under your skin. Remember, it's only the body having a little fit.

3. The runaway eye. This is a twitch of the eyelid. The difficulty with this twitch is that it is visible to other people. A trembling thigh is not obvious in most business conferences. But an eye twitch is, and it tends to put people off. It is particularly offensive if you are a hunchback.

✚ First aid

The general principle of twitch and cramp first aid is "Give the body what it wants." What it wants is either rest or exercise, whichever it hasn't been getting lately. You will have to decide for yourself how you have been mistreating the body.

1. If it's a foot cramp, take the body dancing.

2. Or, stand on one leg.

3. Or, take a hot bath.

4. For eye twitches, spend at least eight hours in a dark room.

5. If all else fails, hold a pistol to the twitching muscle and threaten to shoot it.

Wounds

As a hypochondriac, you are always sick, but you are not always injured. Sooner or later, however, you are bound to suffer some grievous wound, because the world is full of injuries waiting to happen.

There are knives lurking in kitchen drawers, hammers lying on garage shelves, skis waiting in the hall closet. A home workshop that looks to the average person like a nice place to spend an afternoon is in reality a thinly disguised collection of lacerations, avulsions, abrasions, and contusions—not to mention cuts.

Even if you stay out of the workshop, you won't be able to avoid all injury. A potato peeler can do you in. In fact, almost anything can break the skin—paper, paper clips, nail files, a too vigorously wielded pumice stone. A rhinoceros, an elephant, a crocodile—these creatures have skin worthy of the name. We humans might as well have Saran Wrap.

And yet this skin, spread thin to cover the whole body, is all that stands between you and not only injury, but disease. For you must keep in mind that not only do cuts hurt and bleed, they become infected. A nicked finger may not seem like much, but what about blood poisoning, or gangrene? Don't be fooled by a small injury; take them all seriously.

Cuts

A cut is a breach in the body's defensive organ, the skin. Staying

Cuts

healthy and keeping infections out there where they belong, instead of inside your body, is like the war against crime. Just as a broken lock or an open door invites thieves and murderers into your house, so a cut invites infection and disease into your body. Remember, if blood is getting out of the body, other things could get in.

☞ Signs and symptoms

Blood. Cuts invariably bleed.

● Types of cuts

1. Painful. These cuts are small, but cause great suffering. For example: You are planning your summer garden, thinking about what medicinal herbs you would like to plant. In your

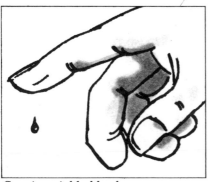

Cuts invariably bleed.

eagerness to see if the seed catalogue has ague-bane, you pull the sharp edge of the cover page between your second and third fingers. This is a painful cut.

2. Ugly. Stay away from these cuts. Nobody likes a messy bleeder. As a self-respecting adult hypochondriac you should stick to clean cuts, painful perhaps, bleeding profusely if that's what the injury calls for, but never ugly. A typical ugly cut is the kind ten-year-old boys get when they fall off a bicycle and land on gravel, asphalt, and broken glass. The result, on arm or knee, is an incomprehensible landscape of blood and skin that tends to put off even sympathetic people.

3. Punctures. These are the ones that cause lockjaw and tetanus. They often don't bleed, and can be almost invisible. (Have a magnifying glass on hand.) But they always have the potential for serious disease. It really doesn't matter how big the wound is,

Cuts

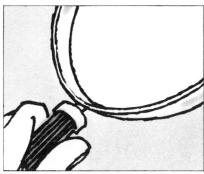

A puncture wound.

or how deep. If something sharp and pointed breaks the skin, you should get a tetanus shot. Remember this simple rhyme: "Long and thin will do you in."

4. "Oh God, I'm going to bleed to death." In painful, ugly, and puncture wounds, blood may dribble, drip, ooze, or well up, like tears. In lacerations, the blood is actually seen to flow, commonly eliciting the comment, "Oh God, I'm going to bleed to death." This is, in fact, a possibility with flowing blood. Immediate action is required.

✗ Causes of cuts

The cause of a cut is often a sharp object, such as a

The ultimate causes of cuts

Cooking pundits. Preparing food is a hazardous occupation, often involving knives, which the pundits who write cooking columns and cookbooks claim should be kept sharp. Sharp knives, they say, cause fewer accidents. This may be true, but the ones they do cause are more bloody. Stick with dull knives. A knife that won't slice a tomato is not going to hurt your finger either.

Spouses. They often put knives in drawers the wrong way, or sharpen them without telling you. (Using dull knife techniques with a sharp knife is particularly dangerous.) Other cuts are caused when the spouse fails to open the mail, thus leaving you wide open to paper cuts.

However, you must be careful about laying blame when you cut yourself. Someone who has just been yelled at for leaving a potato peeler unsheathed is not about to help you bandage your cut.

Children. They may cause cuts by making you furious or frightened. Nothing is more dangerous than chopping garlic just after your three-year-old has expressed intense dislike for you. Is this the Oedipal phase? Is it going well? For him? For you? Thinking these thoughts while you are dicing garlic is a recipe for disaster.

Cuts

knife. This is not the whole story, however. Often the knife was left lying in wait for you. Who left it there? Answer that question and you have the ultimate cause of your cut.

It is obvious that to prevent cuts you should avoid knives, peelers, food processors, razor blades, cans, can openers, sea shells, and twist-off tops. The ultimate causes are harder to trace, but ultimately more important.

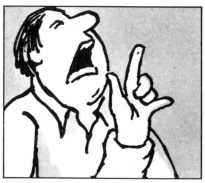

"Honey, I'm bleeding!"

✚ First aid

Blood means an emergency. The reason people faint at the sight of blood is that you're not supposed to see it. It should stay inside the body. If it's outside splashing around, this is a tipoff that something is wrong. Urgent action is required.

1. Except for lacerations, wash cuts out immediately with scalding hot water and soap. This will cause intense pain, and remind you how serious the injury is. It is also likely to make you faint or cry out in an-

guish. This will draw the attention of family or co-workers, who will come to your aid. If no one is in the vicinity, use tepid water.

2. Inspect the cut with great care, making comments like "My God, I really cut myself this time" or "Look at that, it went right through the skin!"

3. Even if it isn't a puncture wound, get a tetanus shot. Always get a tetanus shot.

4. Get someone to help you with the bandage. Use gauze and adhesive tape. For anything that actually bleeds, Band-Aids are too small (save them for pimples and scratches). If no

Cuts

Case history

A woman who had a terrible fear of lockjaw stepped on a tack just as she was about to go on vacation with her husband. Their plane left in five hours. What to do? An hour passed in agonizing indecision as to whether she could risk a long flight and a strange city in her condition.

Finally they decided to go to the emergency room, where she demanded a tetanus shot. The doctor was reluctant. He could not find the point where the tack had allegedly broken the skin. Furthermore, he told her that their records showed that she had been in for a tack attack the year before and had received a tetanus shot at that time. It was too soon to have another one, he said. She insisted. He capitulated, after making her sign a release form.

As soon as she got on the plane, her jaw began to stiffen up. None of the stewardesses knew how long it took a jaw to lock-up permanently, and they seemed unwilling to make an emergency landing. They offered extra fruit juice. The woman, in a panic, kept wiggling her jaw to keep it mobile for the duration of the flight.

She succeeded. However, when she awoke the next morning, her jaw was stiff from all the wiggling, or so her husband contended. She was not entirely convinced that she had not had a mild case of lockjaw, perhaps caused by having had the shot too soon after the last one. Eventually her jaw completely recovered, but she came away from the experience with a fear not only of tetanus, but of tetanus shots.

one is available, make the bandage slightly sloppy. Explain that it is hard to tie a four-in-hand with one hand.

5. When someone sees the bandage and asks you what happened, do not lie. Say, "Oh, nothing, it's just a little cut." Looking at the

size of the bandage, they won't believe you. Instead they will think:

(a) You were seriously injured.

(b) You are brave.

If the blood is flowing

Lacerations require more advanced first aid techniques.

Cuts

1. Never say bleed. Say hemorrhage.

2. Don't use a tourniquet. They look dramatic but they will make your arm fall off.

3. Use pressure to stop the bleeding. You can put pressure on the cut itself, or you can put pressure on your spouse. If you say something like "Honey, I'm bleeding," she will probably come and help you.

If she doesn't, try the children. Often children are not as upset by injuries since they bleed so often themselves, and they may be able to keep a cool head. Pay them off in ice cream. (This may also work for your spouse.) You can also try the neighbors, depending on what they are like. In big cities it is not a good idea to let anyone know that you are bleeding. People may take it as a sign of weakness.

4. Make a really big bandage. (*See* Dressings with Style.)

Preventing infection

The pain and the blood are minor compared to the threat of infection. All cuts require constant attention during the healing process. Colors are the big clues to infection. The first color to watch for is red. If you see red, act quickly. If you wait around, the cut is liable to turn yellow, green, and then black. Anything past yellow means amputation. Inspect the cut every day so that you can follow the healing process. Follow these guidelines:

1. You can't let germs into the cut. But cuts have to breathe. Try to develop a bandaging technique that lets in air but not germs. Failing this, just keep out visible dirt.

2. Change your bandages, and your clothes, daily. Bandages are, after all, the wound's clothes. That's why they are called dressings.

3. Never touch a scab. They are the body's bandages and should remain inviolate.

Contusions

Contusions

Contusions, commonly known as bruises, are inner wounds. The skin stays intact, but underneath the body bleeds, much the way a quiet person responds to an insult. Hypochondriacs, like ripe peaches, bruise easily. The symptoms of a bruise are unmistakable. If you have been contused you will know it.

☞ Signs and symptoms

1. The shout. You are probably a civil person, more given to sighs than bellows. But the initial outrage of a bruise is bound to make you curse. If you hear youself shouting nasty words you have either bruised yourself, or you have La Tourette's syndrome.*

2. The bump. Bruises produce swelling, often dramatic. This is most upsetting. Pain is one thing. It is another to have your body's form altered by egg shapes protruding from shin or scalp, or by fingers swollen out of proportion.

3. The colors. Bruises quickly produce an extraordinary medical rainbow of browns, yellows, blacks, and blues. Like fall foliage, your bruise will change color as its season progresses.

✘ Causes of bruises

The ultimate cause of most bruises is lack of coordination. Fear of the outside world may cause you, like other hypochondriacs, to move in a less than graceful fashion. Being always afraid you are going to bump into something, your tread becomes less sure. And sure enough you do

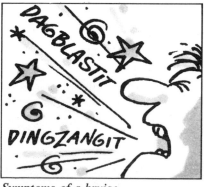

Symptoms of a bruise.

*La Tourette's syndrome is an ailment, apparently neurological, whose victims are given to uncontrollable twitches and outbursts of profanity.

Contusions

bump into things, all sorts of things—tables, chairs, corners, doors, walls. And sometimes you fall.

✚ First aid

Because of the frightening changes bruises cause in the body, it is most important to get other opinions on them. Having other people examine your bruises is crucial.

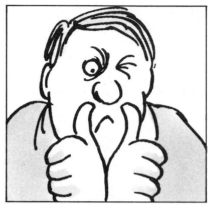

Diagnosing the injury.

1. Say, "What a bump! Can you see it? Feel how big that is."

2. Say, "Look at the color! Did you ever see anything like that? It must have bled a lot internally."

3. Except for one-of-a-kind body parts, like the head, compare the bruised area to its normal counterpart. Have other people aid in the judging and confirm that one finger is, indeed, larger than the other. Also check the shape in case the bone might be broken.

4. Once you have determined that you have a bruise and not a fractured skull or thumb, put ice on it. But be gentle. Remem-

ber, the body has been insulted already. Don't just slap a bag of ice on it. Put the bag in a towel, preferably one that still has some nap.

5. As your outrage fades and the curses subside, you will find yourself left with a smoldering anger. You will be tempted to kick the thing that bruised you. Don't. You will only end up with a stubbed toe, an injury that will bring you to tears. Repress your anger; turn it into depression. Then find a comfortable spot where you can feel sorry for yourself and try to get someone else to feel sorry for you, too.

Dressings with style

When it comes to bandages, the hypochondriac needs to know much more than just how to tape a gauze pad on a laceration. It is important not only to prevent infection and care for the wound, but also to let the bandage speak for the kind of injury you have and the kind of person you are. A good bandage is worth a thousand words.

Your bandage is a signal to the outside world that you have been hurt and deserve some sympathy. With this in mind you will easily learn the proper bandaging techniques. For example, it is obvious that you will get no sympathy for a Band-Aid. A whole-body cast, on the other hand, will move to tears even people who don't like you.

Of course, you have to be reasonable; you can't put a cast on small scrapes. But you can put a lot of gauze and adhesive tape on it. If it's covered with a Band-Aid, it's a scrape; if it's covered with gauze, it's an abrasion. So always have rolls of gauze, gauze pads, and adhesive tape on hand in all different sizes.

Try not to be dull. In dressings, as in dress, fashion is an eyecatcher. Once you've caught their eye, then you can pull people into a discussion of how you got injured, how it feels, and what the chances for gangrene are.

Bandages

Less is not more. More is more. You can never be too rich, too thin, or have too big a bandage.

Bandages

In addition, the dressing should fit your personal style.

Principles of bandaging

1. With an elegant evening dress, use thin adhesive tape. With a dirndl, fat tape works well.

2. If you're a Wall Street type, wear blocky, full-cut, conservative bandages. They should look manly, even if you're a woman.

3. If you are the chef at The Raspberry Sweetbread, you could go for something a bit more elaborate, perhaps a kind of "nouvelle bandage" with dyed tape and a sprig of lemon balm.

4. If you have purple hair and safety pins in your ears, you will probably want to break the rules by wearing no bandage and letting the wound speak for itself. This is a possibility, but remember, a paper cut does not speak with a loud voice. On the other hand, if one of your friends has mugged you, this style is appropriate.

Basic bandage styles

You should feel free to be inventive in your bandaging technique, but start with the classics—the Turban, Pirate's Patch, Gauze Glove, and Roman Legging. With these established styles you can never go wrong. If you follow passing fashions, you are liable to get left short someday. Nothing ruins a good wound faster than a bandage in last season's style.

The turban

Useful for all head wounds, the turban is one of the great triumphs of bandage design. It was originally developed by Indian snake

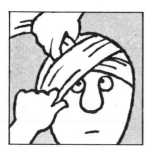 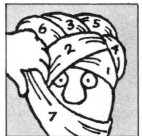 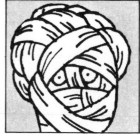

Fig. 1: The turban. For extra security, wrap nose, chin, and mouth.

Bandages

charmers to cover sunburned bald spots and to protect themselves if the cobra leaped at their scalp. It later came to be used to solve the problem of how to get a bandage to stay on your head without sticking adhesive tape to your hair or using a chin strap. The turban has now entered the popular bandage lexicon and can be used for all head injuries. (Fig. 1)

● Wounds

Turban bandages are appropriate for all bumps, bruises, and cuts resulting from:

1. Banging your head on the sharp corner of an open cabinet door.

2. Getting hit with a blackjack by a private eye.

Pirate's patch

The pirate's patch, a stylish eye cover once reserved for serious injuries of the sorts pirates were always performing on one another, has now come into its own. You do not tie a patch yourself, but buy it ready-made. Patches are now available in designer colors, which are particularly appropriate for the summer months. (Fig. 2)

● Wounds

1. Sleeping with your contact lenses in. Requires two patches, a new pair of lenses, and a seeing eye dog. Don't tell anyone what happened. Let them guess.

2. The rubout. When pollen, city air, or cigar smoke causes unbearable itching, you may be able to restrain yourself to the point where you only rub one eye with the heel of your hand. This results in an eye that looks some-

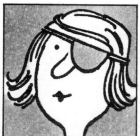 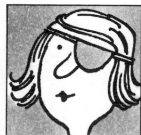 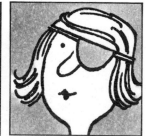

Fig. 2: Pirate's patch. In three colors.

Bandages

thing like a cherry tomato. Cover it.

3. Black eye. In hypochondriacs, this is usually the result of stumbling into a door or being punched out by a doctor. The latter is a clear violation of the Hippocratic oath, as well as assault; it does not, however, qualify as malpractice.

Gauze glove

This looks like a golfer's glove or a driving glove. It just happens to be made of gauze and adhesive tape. This versatile bandage is useful for all hand injuries and goes with any dress style in any season. (Fig. 3)

● **Wounds**

1. Kitchen injuries. If you find that you have sliced, chopped, or diced any part of your hand, use this bandage.

2. Garden injuries. More than fertilizer or watering, gardens demand blisters. The glove will cover them.

3. Also valid for paper cuts and other finger injuries. Finger bandages look silly. It is better to bandage the whole hand.

Roman legging

From the glory that was Rome, a bandage that can truly be described as classic. (Fig. 4)

● **Wounds**

1. Poison ivy. This decidedly unchic rash (not, of course, as déclassé as impetigo) can be greatly increased in importance by the use of the roman legging.

2. Coffee table shin. If you don't watch where you are going (and how can you

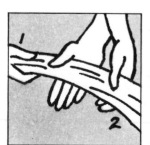
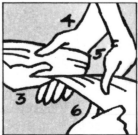
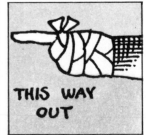

Fig. 3: Gauze glove. Fold 1 over 2; wrap 3 around 5; pull 4 through 6.

Ace bandages

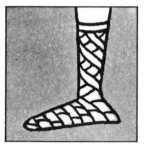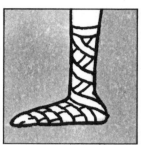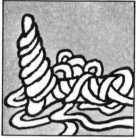

Fig. 4: Roman legging. The Trojan. The Nero. The Caesar.

when you are taking your pulse), seemingly innocent furniture can inflict terrible wounds on your shins.

3. Stubbed toe. Toe bandages are even sillier than finger bandages. Gauze is cheap; feel free to use it to the best effect.

Ace bandages

The great thing about Ace bandages is their sporty look. With an Ace bandage on your knee and a pair of tennis shorts, it is possible to look like a serious athlete without ever having lifted a racquet. If, like most hypochondriacs, you want to be part of the world at large but find participation somewhat frightening, Ace bandages are a godsend.

Sprains, strains, and aches are the injuries for which Ace bandages are used. You will have plenty of these. It is just as easy to twist an ankle running for a bus as it is trying to score a soccer goal. And you know what can happen on the exercycle, or trying to keep up with a child in the park. You may even be injured in the actual practice of a sport. You only have to play tennis once to hurt your knee. Then you can have a safe season of adjusting your Ace bandage while you drink gin and tonics at a courtside table.

One of the attractions of Ace bandages is that they don't tear your body hair off the way adhesive tape does. But they do have some drawbacks.

1. Wrapped too tightly, an Ace bandage can completely cut off the circulation in leg or arm, resulting fairly quickly in gangrene.

2. Wrapped too loosely an

Casts

Ace bandage looks like a support stocking that is falling down.

3. It is next to impossible to wrap an Ace bandage that is neither too tight nor too loose.

Casts

A broken bone is a no-nonsense injury. Even most health chauvinists will admit it if they have snapped a fibula. Consequently, the dressing for a broken bone—a cast—has enormous cachet in the non-hypochondriacal world. The medical value of a cast lies in the immobilization of the bone to encourage healing, but the value to the hypochondriac is that a cast is the kind of badge that encourages self-respect.

There is no agonizing self-doubt about whether there is really something wrong with you. And you don't have to put up with a lot of sarcastic remarks the way you do with cardiac arrhythmias. No other bandage will do this for you. Even with a sling, suspicious people may think that you rigged it yourself. No one doubts a cast.

Furthermore, a cast is a social as well as a medical status symbol if you attain it in the pur-

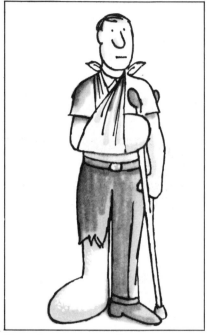

Casts have great cachet.

suit of a dangerous and fashionable sport, such as skiing. As a hypochondriac, you will probably have broken your leg stepping off a curb. But nobody has to know. You can feign a stoic unwillingness to talk about the injury, and let people imagine what they will.

Some rules about casts:

1. In case of any injury—sprain, strain, or bruise—get an X-ray. You never know when a bone might have cracked.

2. Insist on a cast. If the doctor proposes a sling, tell him

Casts

you are clumsy and don't trust yourself not to fall and smash the arm again.

3. The bigger the cast, the more you should play down the injury. You can describe a hairline wrist fracture as a "bad break," but if your whole arm is in a cast, refer to your injury as a "small accident."

4. Don't have people sign your cast. This shows disrespect for the injury. Claim the bone is too tender. In this era of decorated casts, the stark whiteness of yours will make it stand out all the more. And people will feel particularly sorry for you because they will think that in addition to suffering from a broken leg, you don't have any friends.

5. When the cast is removed, the injury is not over. Now, while the memory of the cast is still fresh, you may safely use a sling. Or, if the injury was to the leg, wear crutches for a while. Then limp and refuse to carry groceries for months afterward.

Shock and disappointment

Shock is the body's response to a severe injury. Common physical causes of shock are car accidents and gunshot wounds. The cardinal characteristic of shock in these cases is that you will be completely incapacitated. Someone else will have to take care of you.

But psychological trauma can also cause shock. This is the kind of shock that you should be worried about—a debilitating physical response to upsetting events. Not only do you become depressed, so do all your bodily functions. Disappointment is a similar lowering of body functions that is less severe.

As a hypochondriac you will know the feelings that accompany shock, although you may not have had a medical name for them. When your wife and your cardiologist run off together, leaving you completely alone, the illness that comes over you is shock. When your husband remembers your birthday, but gives you potholders, that is disappointment. Non-hypochondriacs do not believe that physical illness accompanies such events. Therefore you will have to provide your own medical attention.

Shock

There are many kinds of shock. The most common are romantic, occupational, and tennis shock.

Shock

✗ Causes

Bad events.

Examples are:

1. In the midst of a heated argument with your new girlfriend, you say, "It's important for me to share my feelings with you." She responds by shouting, "Your feelings? All you ever feel is sick. Who needs to share that?" Suddenly, you feel sick.

2. You overhear your boss asking someone who you are. A wave of nausea comes over you.

3. You lose a club tennis tournament in a dismal final match in which a man ten years your junior runs you into the ground. You become acutely aware of how bald you are, and how much hair he has. Your heart falters.

Good events.

Doctors have shown that stress accompanies good events as well as bad. Getting divorced is known to cause stress. So does getting married. Either can cause shock. Other examples are:

1. The woman of your dreams, who bears a frightening resemblance to Bo Derek, invites you to her apartment for some Harvey's Bristol Cream.

2. You are promoted. You wonder if, as an assistant branch manager, you will now be a target for the Red Brigades.

☞ Signs and symptoms

1. A sudden awareness of your own mortality. Not that you are ever unaware of it, but shock brings the fear of death to the fore. Usually it comes in the form of a chill. Often you believe you are dying at that moment.

2. Palpitations and arrhythmias. A rapid, weak pulse. You will notice this immediately after the awareness of mortality strikes, when you take your pulse to see if your heart is failing.

3. Weakness. If you try to make a fist, you will find that you don't have the strength.

4. Whole-body nausea. This occurs when not only

Shock

your stomach but your arms, legs, and face feel sick. You doubt that you can go on.

✚ First aid

The first principle of shock first aid is to stay warm. The second principle is not to be alone.

Body temperature, and comfort

1. Wrap yourself in blankets and sweaters. Put the soft, worn cotton blankets next to the skin, and the warmth-giving woolen blankets on the outside. Cover everything but your mouth and nose. You need to be able to breathe and to consume your favorite foods.

2. Have someone take care of you. If the person you would usually ask to make hot chocolate for you is the one who caused the shock, put a dog in your lap.

3. Take your temperature. Fever has nothing to do with shock, but having a thermometer in your mouth will make you feel more secure.

Body position

1. For romantic shock, sit in a rocking chair and rock back and forth hugging yourself. This works for divorce also, and for certain kinds of good news shock. This is the procedure to follow when you realize that the woman of your dreams is so healthy you are afraid she might injure you. You would much rather have a nurse.

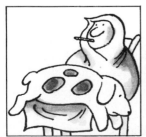 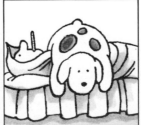 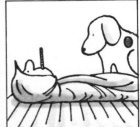

Shock first aid (from left): Rocking, reclining, prostrate.

Disappointment

2. Semi-reclining. This is the classic couch position, useful for medium-level shock. If it helps, imagine that your psychiatrist is behind you. This may just set you up for disappointment, however, if you suddenly remember he is not there.

3. Prostrate. For severe shock, such as when you learn you really do have high blood pressure. Lie flat on your back on the floor wrapped up like a mummy, with a pillow under your head. Meditate on what it is to be an invalid.

Fluids

1. Drink ginger ale. This is the hypochondriac's main sustenance during shock, colds, and other periods of debilitation.

Disappointment

Disappointment is mild shock tinged with melancholia. It is not as physically debilitating as shock, but does require medical attention.

✗ Causes

1. Your dream woman invites you to lunch so you can help her pick out a birthday gift for her boyfriend, who plays rugby.

2. Your boss speaks to you for the first time in weeks. But all he says is hello.

3. You win the tennis tournament. But you are still bald.

☞ Signs and symptoms

Disappointment produces a vague feeling of unworthiness. Physically, this is usually expressed in the symptoms of degenerative disease.

1. Your joints ache. You wonder if you have arthritis. You imagine that soon you will be too ill for romance even if it does come your way.

2. Your depression seems to you the result of a disturbance in your brain, probably a tumor. But you are too depressed to see a doctor.

3. You get out of breath easily. You have pains in

Disappointment

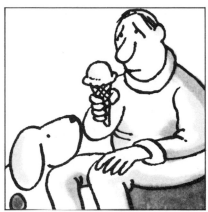

Disappointment.

your chest. You suspect angina.

✚ First aid

For disappointment, making several doctor's appointments is the first step. Force yourself to do it even if you don't want to. This will help shake off your depression. You should see an orthopedic man, a cardiologist, a neurologist, and your own internist.

In the meantime, follow these procedures:
1. Wrap yourself in blankets, but not as tightly as for shock, and use only cotton ones. If you are only mildly disappointed, a comfortable sweater and a friendly pair of slippers will do.

2. Keep the dog off your lap. This will only make you feel silly. Have it put its head on your knee.

3. Don't use the prostrate position. With disappointment you have to carry on bravely in the face of infirmity. If you do this well enough, you may get unsolicited sympathy, which, for a hypochondriac, is like winning the World Series

4. Have ice cream with your ginger ale.

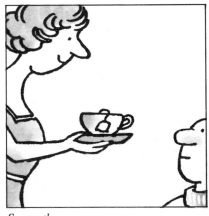

Sympathy.

Cold comfort

Never take a cold lightly. Colds can worsen into pneumonia. They can lower your resistance and lay you wide open to swollen glands and strep throat. They share some of the same symptoms with big league diseases like bubonic plague. And don't forget that while doctors may have eradicated smallpox from the face of the earth, they haven't been able to do anything about colds. You have to respect any disease that is harder to conquer than smallpox.

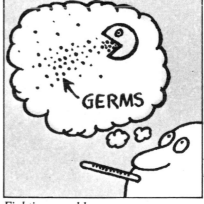
Fighting a cold.

This respect will be increased if you think of what is actually happening during a cold. Viruses, small bits of DNA with protein coats, have no cells or cell machinery of their own. So they hijack the cells of innocent people like yourself, and use your cell machinery to reproduce. No wonder you feel sick.

When your body is being held hostage by an army of these submicroscopic terrorists, this is not the time to go on about your business saying, "Oh, it's just a cold." You must rest, build up your body's own resources, and conserve your strength so that you

Colds

can fight the viruses. You can help the body by cheering on your immune system. This bodily defense system is beyond true conscious control, but there is some evidence that a fighting spirit can actually help recovery. You must visualize the immune system and imagine that you are sending it into battle:

Out go your white blood cells—lymphocytes—to attack the invaders. Envision these killer cells as SWAT teams stopping the hijackers. Or if you have a taste for video games, imagine lymphocytes as little Pac-Men gobbling up the viruses.

If you are on the political left, and abhor SWAT teams and video game frivolity, you might want to think of the viruses as FBI agents who have illegally broken into your home in flagrant violation of the Bill of Rights. In this case the immune system becomes the ACLU.

Colds

You won't know how to fight a cold if you don't know you have it. Keep a close watch for these symptoms.

1. In the first stage you will feel that someone is sweeping your sinuses with a stiff-bristled broom.

2. The next stage is characterized by three symptoms:

(a) The sweeping feeling goes and you wake up one morning convinced that every space in your nose and head has been packed with grouting compound. This puts the tasks of eating and breathing in competition for the use of the mouth, and sometimes makes the old adage to "feed a cold" seem like a sure recipe for asphyxiation.

(b) You find that your weight has doubled and that it is impossible to make quick movements. It takes a great effort to move at all.

(c) The viruses have also invaded your brain cells, resulting in a precipitous drop in IQ and temporary dyslexia.

3. In the third stage the cold moves to the chest. The death rattle makes its first appearance. When someone asks how you are,

Colds

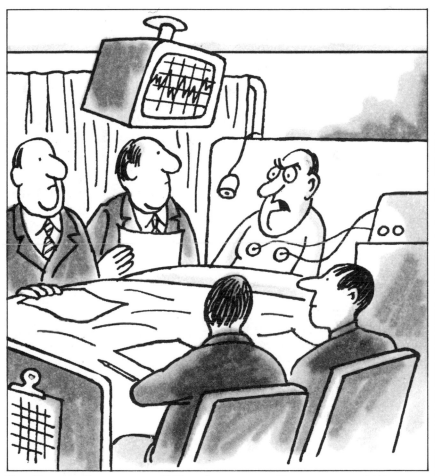

THE HEALTH CHAUVINIST. *"What do you mean Harris is out sick?"*

you don't answer right
away, you cough first.
Then you croak, with a
pained face, "I'm all right."

✗ Causes

1. Wet feet. (This also
causes rheumatic fever.)
2. Winter.
3. Health chauvinism. This
is the biggest cause of
colds, as well as a major
source of unhappiness for
all hypochondriacs. Health

Colds

chauvinists believe that it is a character flaw to catch a cold at all, and unforgivable spinelessness to admit it. They are the people who are always saying, "I never get sick." Consequently, while the sick hypochondriac stays at home keeping his germs to himself, the health chauvinist is out in public spreading cold virus as if it were Christmas cheer. He (or she, health chauvinism knows no sexual boundaries) seems not to notice his cough, his runny nose, the washboard scrape in his chest when he breathes. A health chauvinist with plague would come to work on a Monday morning in August, and kiss you hello.

Don't try to convince health chauvinists that they are sick. Avoid them. It is not possible to be friends with them anyway.

✚ First aid

Doctors do not take care of colds. They try to give the impression that colds are not real diseases and are not worthy of their attention. This is a medical con game. Colds are perfectly good diseases. It's the doctors who aren't so great. When you do get a cold, don't bother calling a physician. Treat your cold yourself. Follow these instructions.

1. Stay home from work.
(a) When you first call in sick, use the Voice of the Dead. Call early in the morning, when your throat and chest have not yet cleared. You won't even have to say that you are not coming in. The receptionist will usually respond to your hoarse hello by saying, "Who is this?" When you tell her, she will say, "You sound awful."
(b) The Health Chauvinist Boss. These men and women consider it an act of disloyalty when one of their subordinates comes down with a cold. They know, however, that it is socially unacceptable, and probably illegal, to insist that people come to work when they are sick. If you work for one of these peo-

Colds

ple, you may avoid recrimination by putting the decision as to whether you come to work in their hands. Say, "I've got a fever and a sore throat and I'm coughing blood, but I'll be glad to come in if you need me."

2. Treat yourself right.

When you have a cold, comfort is all important. You must set yourself up in a sickroom with food, drink, entertainment, and medication all at hand.

(a) Food. Certain foods are appropriate for cold victims and others are not. You want safe, friendly foods that will make you feel taken care of. You don't want demanding foods, even if you might like them at some other time. And you don't want angry foods such as pepperoni.

(b) Drink. Similar to food. Don't drink anything physiologically or psychologically demanding.

(c) The sofa. It is impos-

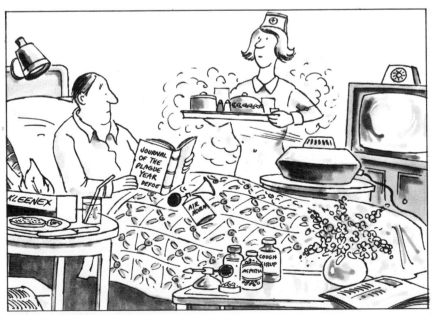

Outfit your sickroom for comfort.

Colds

The right stuff

The Right Foods	The Wrong Foods
English muffins	Liver
Marmalades	Artichokes
Ice cream	Sea slugs
Shortbread	Haggis*

The Right Drinks	The Wrong Drinks
Ginger ale	Liver and egg health shake
Tea	Clamato juice
Fresh orange juice	Gatorade
Ice water	Kumiss**

The Right TV	The Wrong TV
"As the World Turns"	"The CBS Morning News"
"I Love Lucy"	"The CBS Evening News"
"Gilligan's Island"	"Quincy"
"The Mary Tyler Moore Show"	Anything on public television

The Right Authors	The Wrong Authors
Agatha Christie	Dostoevsky
P. G. Wodehouse	Henry James
Mark Twain	Gertrude Stein
Daniel Defoe***	Kafka

*Spicy Scottish dish made of internal parts of a sheep stuffed into the sheep's stomach.
**Fermented camel's milk. Popular with Asian nomads.
***His *Journal of the Plague Year* will always give you a lift.

sible to be comfortable without a sofa. A bed is too clinical and a chair too unfriendly. You must set yourself up on a couch with a hand-knit afghan, preferably made by your grandmother, to keep you warm. An old-fashioned, overstuffed couch is best. Modular furniture is out. As is anything made from

The flu

leather and chrome. If you have a taste for steel and chrome, save it for the kitchen. (*See* The Med-Tech Kitchen.)

(d) Television. You can't spend all your time brooding about those viruses in your cells. You need to be distracted. Daytime television was made for this. You will feel that since you are sick you are allowed to suspend all critical judgment, and you will thus be able to laugh freely at "Gilligan's Island," one of life's simplest pleasures.

(e) Books. Watching television all day long will upset your stomach. You should spend some time reading. Stay away from books with long sentences, subtle insights, and depressing subjects.

(f) Get enough rest. Sleep at least 10 hours a night. Take a morning nap, after the paper and the first chapter of *Jeeves Goes to Boston*, and an evening snooze after "Mary Tyler Moore." Try never to become fully awake.

(g) Take the right medica-tion. Find a good cold pill that dries up your nose and makes you pleasantly drowsy. Don't drink alcohol with it, and never mix any medication with Clamato juice.

Cold cousins

There are other diseases that are related to colds and receive much the same treatment (they all require comfort) but are somewhat more serious. The primary one is the flu. Others are pneumonia, bronchitis, and the hypochondriac's horror, laryngitis.

Some of these diseases are accompanied by fevers. One thing to remember about fevers is that the rule to feed a cold and starve a fever is wrong. You should feed every ailment except food poisoning. When you don't eat it is you that starves, not the fever.

The flu

The flu is more severe than a cold, although it shares some of the same symptoms. One thing to remember is that people have died from the flu. But this doesn't

Pneumonia

mean you should get flu shots.

Hypochondriacs always refuse to get flu shots because they are afraid the shots might actually give them the flu, or cause Guillain-Barré syndrome, which results in a form of paralysis. This syndrome killed several elderly people during the recent swine flu scare. Of course, hypochondriacs always end up getting the flu and wishing that they had gotten the shots.

☞ Signs and symptoms

1. Muscle aches and sore skin. It is impossible to be comfortable in any bed, couch, or chair. This aspect of the illness is particularly trying on the families of hypochondriacs. As a hypochondriac you should try to limit your moaning to a level that allows you to express how bad you feel, but does not completely alienate those around you.
2. A real, honest-to-goodness fever. All your thermometers agree. You know you are sick.

✚ First aid

The same as for a cold. Just stay out of work longer.

Pneumonia

☞ Signs and symptoms

A painful cough, high fever, and delirium.

✚ First aid

1. See a doctor. You can't fool around with pneumonia. In addition to your prescriptions, be sure to have him give you a signed statement that you have had pneumonia. This is important for showing to other people, who will never believe you if you don't have it.
2. Stay out of work for at least two weeks. You may want to have a decorator in to create a permanent sickroom. Once you have had pneumonia, there is no way of telling how long convalescence will take, or when the disease will strike again.

Bronchitis

This is a serious inflammation of the bronchial tubes, much feared by hypochondriacs. It can be acute or chronic.

Bronchitis

How to work a thermometer

The thermometer is the hypochondriac's most important tool. It serves not only to determine whether you have a fever, but also to give you the sense of security that comes from knowing that you are monitoring your bodily functions.

A thermometer also provides a solid connection to reality. As a hypochondriac, you may be drawn so far into an illness that you don't know when you have recovered. You can take your temperature to find out if you are still sick.

And finally, the thermometer is a diagnostic tool; it helps you determine what kind of illness you have. A low fever or a temperature below normal is a sign of a "low-grade infection"—a cold or a "bug." A high temperature may mean that you have contracted one of the cold's closest cousins—the flu. A thermometer won't tell you exactly what you've got, but if you feel bad and are not sure whether it is depression, anxiety, or malaria, the thermometer will at least narrow your choices.

Some thermometer guidelines

1. Keep four or five thermometers on hand. You will be safe if you lose or break one or two, and you can test them against one another. Thermometers are notoriously inaccurate, so you should never trust just one reading.

2. Oral thermometers are perfectly adequate. Even hypochondria has its limits.

3. Always keep a thermometer in your mouth for at least 10 minutes. Try not to breathe through your mouth during this time. The cooling effect of air passing over the thermometer may invalidate the reading.

4. Carry a thermometer with you wherever you go.

☞ **Signs and symptoms**

1. Acute. A bad cough.
2. Chronic. A bad cough that lasts for more than a week.

✚ **First aid**

Never go out in cold weather—for the rest of your life.

Laryngitis

Laryngitis

👉 Signs and symptoms

1. You are unable to complain.
2. Family members show symptoms of relief and delight. They refuse to call a doctor or give you any medicine. They also will not lip-read or look at notes that you have written. They pretend not to see when you frantically wave your arms in a desperate quest for ginger ale.

✚ First aid

1. Plot revenge. Write down everything you feel so that you can tell everyone about it, over and over, once you get your voice back.
2. Buy an air horn. This will get their attention.

The breath of life

Any training in first aid must include expertise in breathing. As a bodily function there is no underestimating its importance. And yet, breathing is normally not within our conscious control. This makes sense, of course, because someone has to keep the body breathing while you are asleep or thinking of something else. But the situation would be terrifying except that there are channels of intra-body communication that allow you to override the brain's automatic pilot. You can take over your own breathing.

This is necessary because the automatic breathing process can be interrupted or halted by a number of occurrences, from disease to strangulation. Then you have to do your own breathing, which is not as simple as it seems. If you take over too soon and too vigorously, you hyperventilate. If you don't take over when necessary, the results are obvious.

As a hypochondriac, you may be tempted to try to do your own breathing all the time, just to be on the safe side. This is overdoing it. It is also exhausting. What you need to do is to learn how and when to do your own breathing. This essential first aid technique is not at all complicated and no equipment is required. Just remember, "In goes the good air; out goes the bad."

Artificial respiration

Artificial respiration

1. Clear your airway. Do this by moving your tongue to one side with your finger. Try not to choke yourself, this will only complicate matters. (Fig. 1)

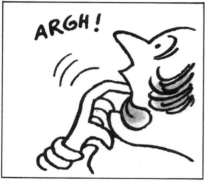

Fig. 1

2. Use your chest and abdominal muscles to squeeze your

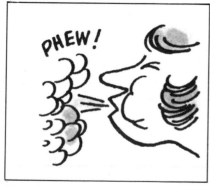

Fig. 2

lungs, blowing air out your mouth. (Fig. 2)

3. Use the same muscle to expand your chest, opening up your lungs and pulling in air. You

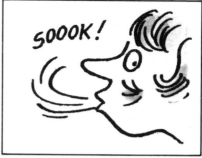

Fig. 3

will feel the air rush through your cheeks. (Fig. 3)

4. Do this procedure once every five seconds.

Warning: use artificial respiration only when necessary. If you panic and use it when it is not necessary, it will cause hyperventilation.

Hyperventilation

Hyperventilation afflicts nervous people—many of whom are hypochondriacs—who are too quick to take over from the automatic pilot and run their own breathing. Faced with something

Hyperventilation

that makes them anxious, they are overcome with the fear that they are not getting enough air and they start doing a lot of unnecessary extra breathing, thus overloading the brain with oxygen.

The brain, afraid it will burn out from excess oxygen, shuts everything down, which is when the hyperventilator faints.

☞ Signs and symptoms
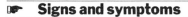

Heavy breathing—your own.

✗ Causes

Anything that can make you nervous can cause hyperventilation. Common causes of hyperventilation are:
1. Falling in love.
2. Thinking about falling in love.
3. Not falling in love.

✚ First aid

1. Breathe into a bag. Do not worry how silly you look. If you are embarrassed about being the sort of anxious, fearful, incompetent person who hyperventilates, you can claim to be sniffing glue. (Fig. 4)

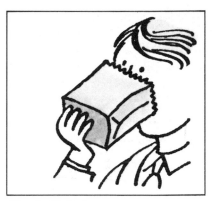

Fig. 4: Right bag.

2. Do not use a plastic dry cleaner's bag. (Fig. 5)

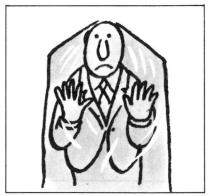

Fig. 5: Wrong bag.

Inability to breathe

Sometimes, meteorological or social conditions seem to steal the oxygen from the air. You then

Inability to breathe

find that you "can't breathe." In fact, what has happened is that the automatic pilot is so appalled by what is going on that it ceases to operate properly.

You should learn to diagnose these situations so you know when to give artificial respiration.

✗ Meteorological causes

1. Overheated air of the sort commonly found in buses and old ladies' apartments.

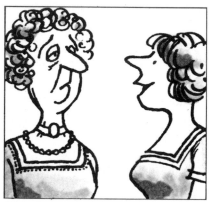

Fig. 6: "Thistake it 's meest! And after meath the dulwich."

2. Too many people in a small space breathing up all the available air. (There are social complications to crowding. In figuring how much air is being sucked away from you, one relative counts for five strangers or 10 friends.)

✗ Social causes

1. Family parties where your great-aunt, who can't remember that you're not married, keeps asking you why you don't have any children. To everything you say, she answers, "What?"

2. Bringing home a boyfriend and having your fa-

ther discourse at length on the principles of medieval cartography.

3. Being brought to a boyfriend's home and having his mother say:
(a) "You're Jewish?"
or
(b) "You're not Jewish?"

☞ Signs and symptoms

1. The feeling that somebody is stealing your air, on purpose.

2. The sensation of breathing shredded wheat.

3. Tightness in the chest, pain, and the overwhelming desire to steal someone else's air.

Choking

✚ First aid

1. Find the radiator in the room. Turn off the heat, and open the window.
2. Take the emotional initiative. Before anyone has a chance to speak, announce your ethnic and religious roots, your politics, and your sexual preference. This will either clear the air, or take their breath away. Your own breathing will remain unimpaired.
3. Recite sections of *Finnegans Wake* to your aunt in response to all her questions. (Fig. 6)
4. Take the physical initiative, and give yourself artificial respiration.

Choking

Choking is a special case under the larger category of Inability to Breathe. It comes on suddenly and is unmistakable to the person who is choking. It also has a specific cure. By now, everyone has seen the posters on the walls in restaurants showing a choking victim being wrestled to the ground and punched in the stomach by others performing the first aid technique called the Heimlich maneuver.*

The Heimlich maneuver is an effective procedure. For it to work, however, someone else has to be there when you choke. And you have to be of a trusting nature. Many hypochondriacs, on being attacked by dinner companions while they are choking, might not interpret this as an attempt to help. If you choke when you are alone, or you don't trust others to perform violent pseudomedical procedures on you, you need to know what to do for yourself. First, you must recognize that you are choking.

☞ Signs and symptoms

1. A sudden cessation of breathing. This is different from the feeling that someone has swiped all the oxygen from the air, and left you to breathe dust and ashes. In this case, no air at all comes in and none goes out.
2. A tight feeling in the throat. If, for example, you

*Heimlich is a secular alternative to St. Blaise, the patron saint of choking victims. The St. Blaise maneuver involves going to church on St. Blaise's day, and having your throat blessed. You can, of course, use both maneuvers.

Sleep apnea

were having a stroke and your breathing nerves had been knocked out, you wouldn't have this sensation. It is a sure indication of choking.

3. Appalled looks on the faces of people around you.

✗ Causes

1. Fish bones. This is how St. Blaise made his name, by saving a choking victim.
2. Talking, and breathing, with your mouth full. This lets a bit of food go down the wrong way. Food headed for the lungs instead of the stomach invariably causes choking. The danger of this happening is the reason table manners were invented.

✚ First aid

If you are sure you are choking:

1. Extend both arms to reach around your body from the back and hold yourself tightly with the fists placed at the solar plexus. (If you are too fat to be able to get your arms around yourself, try No. 3 below.)

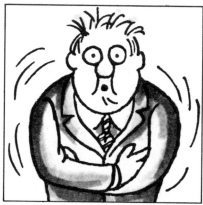

Fig. 7: The solitary Heimlich.

2. Pull in sharply with your fists, several times. (Fig. 7) Or,
3. If you can't Heimlich yourself in the classic fashion, try using a couch or some well-padded corner. Rest your solar plexus on the corner and push forward, several times sharply. Do not take a running start. You want to stop choking, not impale yourself on a sofa.

Sleep apnea

Sleep apnea is a little-known respiratory syndrome much feared by hypochondriacs. Its most frightening aspect is that you may not know that you have it. In this syndrome, while you are asleep,

Sleep apnea

your breathing stops. Normally the build-up of carbon dioxide in the blood stimulates the respiratory center of the brain. In sleep apnea this process fails. In plain language, the automatic pilot falls asleep on the job.

You may awake gasping for air, your breathing may spontaneously recover, or you may never wake up again. Sleep apnea can be fatal.

☞ Signs and symptoms

1. Waking with a start. If as you begin to fall asleep, you find yourself thrown into wakefulness by the feeling that you are being choked, either you have sleep apnea or your bedmate is not trustworthy.
2. Feeling tired in the morning. This could be because you haven't been breathing enough while you are asleep.

✚ First aid

1. Don't sleep alone. Have your bedmate wake you if he or she notices that you have stopped breathing.
2. Don't sleep with anyone you don't trust.
3. Don't sleep.

Case history

A man whose wife was an insufferable (so he thought) hypochondriac became involved in an argument with her over medical bills. He contended that three electrocardiograms in a month by three different doctors was excessive. She responded by asking him if he wanted her to die.

This set off a rather nasty argument. The woman was by far the better arguer, having a vast amount of medical knowledge to draw on. The man finally started pointing out symptoms she had that she hadn't noticed. He asked her if she had ever realized that she might have giardiasis, a parasitic infection that is usually symptomless in adults. When she began to quaver, he administered the coup de grâce.

"And another thing," he said. "I see you when you fall asleep. And you don't know it, but you have sleep apnea." This attack took her breath away. It also sent her to the doctor immediately. The man realized then, that in terms of medical bills—which had started the whole argument—his victory was a Pyrrhic one.

Poisons

The average person associates poisons with medieval court intrigue or Agatha Christie novels. The hypochondriac knows the truth, that ordinary everyday life is saturated with poisons, and that the worst are the ones you least suspect, such as the leaves of tomato plants.* If you can't trust a tomato, what can you trust?

Nothing. You should suspect anything that you can breathe, eat, drink, or touch. Paints and varnishes are obvious, because they smell poisonous. Food is the worst of all, because on the surface it seems like something you might want to eat. And yet it can harbor dangerous bacteria. Some foods, such as mushrooms, can be innately poisonous. Shellfish can poison you in three different ways, the worst of

which results in paralysis. And so-called wild foods, harvested from the woods, are deadly if you pick the wrong plant. You have to ask yourself, if wild food is so good, why is Euell Gibbons dead?

The household is also poisonous. You may, for instance, have become giddy while waxing the floor. Quite reasonably you concluded that the fumes from the wax were poisoning you. Reeling, and trying to stay conscious, you telephoned the local poison control center. No doubt they were not sympathetic.

Hypochondriacs are being poisoned like this all the time,

*If you are a beginning gardener, you may need help in interpreting what you are growing. Who knows what part of a kohlrabi is edible, and how to eat it? Get a field guide to garden vegetables, and use it diligently.

Food poisoning

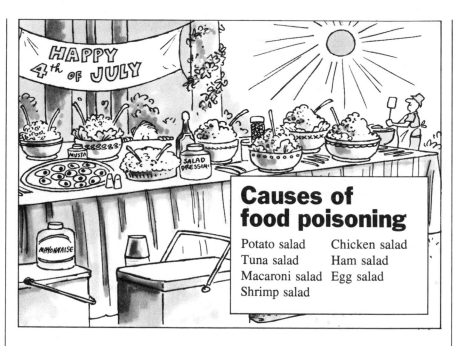

Causes of food poisoning

Potato salad   Chicken salad
Tuna salad   Ham salad
Macaroni salad Egg salad
Shrimp salad

often by themselves. You won't die from floor wax, but it can frighten and embarrass you. To prevent this from happening, you should learn your poisons, and avoid them.

Food poisoning

Food itself is not usually poisonous, although there are exceptions. But food does breed the bacteria that cause food poisoning. Some foods are worse than others, but nothing is completely safe; consequently, eating is never without risk.

Some people even eat foods they know are poisonous. The Japanese are fond of a kind of blowfish that, if improperly prepared, will kill you. Even if properly prepared the fish retains some of its natural poisons, and causes a mild "high." Devotees of this dish seem to enjoy the risk.

For hypochondriacs, it is not necessary to eat exotic foods to flirt with death. They feel they are taking a big gamble every time they eat a tuna fish sandwich.

Food poisoning

✖ Causes

1. Eating in restaurants.* Restaurant kitchens are game preserves for poisonous bacteria. As long as there are restaurants these organisms will never become extinct. (Fast-food restaurants are an excption, since the "food" they serve is made from petrochemicals, and bacteria can't live in it.)

2. Fourth of July picnics. The deviled eggs, potato salad, and tuna fish served at these affairs are more dangerous than the holiday traffic. Nothing strikes fear into the heart of a hypochondriac—and well it should—more than a bowl of potato salad sitting in the sun. It is a bomb, waiting to go off.

It is the mayonnaise that attracts the bacteria that cause food poisoning. When mayonnaise is in the hot sun it becomes deadly. Foods with mayonnaise in them can be eaten safely only in air-conditioned rooms where the light is not too bright.

☞ Signs and symptoms

1. Queasiness. A feeling that your body, particularly in the area of your stomach, doesn't quite fit you anymore. You have a sense of imminent catastrophe.
2. Nausea. Sweating. Catastrophe seems certain.
3. Catastrophe. You are also racked by chills and fever. You want to die.

✚ First aid

There is very little you can do to stop food poisoning. It has to run its course. You can make it go more quickly if you don't fight it. Trying to hang on to a dinner that you know you are going to lose is misplaced perseverance. It only makes things worse in the end.

Food poisoning is always frightening and depressing. Sometimes when uncontrollable chills strike, in between bouts of throwing up, you may be tempted to weep. If this is so:

*You can also catch typhoid at a restaurant. Before you eat anywhere, look for people who might be carriers.

Bc tulism

1. Wrap yourself in a warm blanket. Have someone hug you during the chills.
2. Plan a review of the restaurant where you ate, describing what the food did to you. If you really suffer, you could always type it up and tape it to their window.

ulism

Botulism is different from food poisoning because it doesn't just make you ill. It kills you. The botulin toxin is produced by bacteria that grow in canned food.

Some people just make sure that they don't eat the brands or batches that have been recalled. Why take the chance? As a hypochondriac it is easier to give up all canned mushrooms than worry for the rest of your life whether this can or that will kill you.

The same goes for salmon and cold potato soup. In fact, it is easier never to eat anything that comes from a can. If you do, watch for these symptoms.

☞ Signs and symptoms

1. Vomiting.
2. Paralysis of the eyes.
3. Loss of voice.

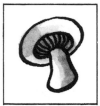
Safe.

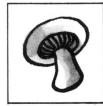
Poison.

✚ First aid

If you have these symptoms, you have been poisoned by botulism. It is now too late to call a doctor since you can't read the telephone book and have lost your voice. There is no first aid possible.

Chemical poisons

Almost everything made by man, from lighter fluid to nail polish, is poisonous. It would be best never to use anything that has the word *"Caution"* on its label. If this is not possible, concentrate on the two most poisonous substances known to man—insect sprays and household cleaners.

1. Insect sprays. Aphid sprays, ant and roach sprays, wasp and hornet sprays are part of any home's defense budget. All

Chemical poisons

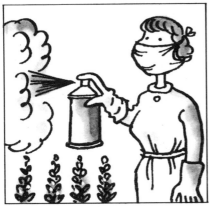

Aphid spray protection.

are poisonous to people, no matter what the label says. Follow these precautions:

(a) Always wear rubber gloves and a mask.

(b) Never spray your lunch.

(c) Never spray in the room you are in.

2. Household cleaners. All of these are also poisonous to people. The worst are oven cleaners. Cleaning an oven is roughly as dangerous as decontaminating Three Mile Island. Follow these precautions:

(a) Hire a cleaning woman. If this bothers your conscience, or your pocketbook, the best policy is:

(b) Rent an apartment and move to a new one when the oven gets too dirty to use. Or, for a long-term solution:

(c) Marry a health chauvinist. They don't particularly like cleaning ovens, but if you whine a bit about how the oven cleaner causes cancer, brain lesions, and dizziness, they get so irritated that they rush off and clean the oven just to show you it's not so bad. This is the only constructive use of health chauvinism.

☞ Signs and symptoms

Household cleaners and bug sprays have the same effects, for some reason. In fact, in a pinch you can spray oven cleaner on ants. It will kill them. Bug spray, however, does not cut through grease very well.

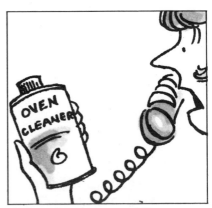

Calling "poison central."

Chemical poisons

1. Headache. All odd-smelling poisonous fumes cause headaches.

2. Sore throat and lungs. You can feel where the long molecules have damaged the sensitive internal tissues.

✚ First aid

1. Do not call the poison control center unless you have actually swallowed the oven cleaner. Those people are very picky about what constitutes poisoning.

2. Read the label. (Be sure to put on gloves and a mask first.) This will tell you what to do in case of poisoning. Do everything except call the poison control center.

3. Have someone sit with you to observe any changes. Failing this, look in the mirror frequently. If your skin changes color, or you can't make it to the mirror, you can then call the poison control center without fear of reprisal.

Kitchen surgery

Any doctor will tell you that only a doctor can perform surgery. Nonsense. In the old days, barbers used to do surgery. The inept few still do. And there are many doctors who would do the world a great favor if they turned to cutting hair.

And you, too, should learn how to do surgery. Of course, if you need a coronary bypass, or a brain tumor removed, you need a bona fide surgeon. Such operations are beyond the scope of kitchen surgery. But slivers are not.

And slivers are nothing to laugh at. Not only can they cause great pain and dangerous infections, they have been a great spur over the ages to technical development. Slivers are responsible for the development of rugs, lino-

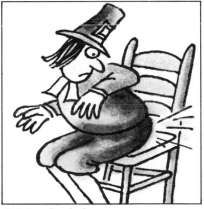

Origin of upholstery.

leum, upholstered furniture, gloves, and plastic toilet seats. In fact, some observers believe the entire plastics industry was spawned by a desire to eliminate slivers. Slivers are painful, they cause infection, and no one wants to have a foreign body in the body.

If you get a sliver, you have

Slivers

two choices. You can go to the emergency room, where you will be charged an arm and a leg—no matter where the sliver is. Or you can learn to do kitchen surgery. Not only will you save money by operating on yourself, you can be sure that your surgeon has your interests at heart. Once you have learned kitchen surgery for slivers, you will find that the same techniques can be applied to trimming hangnails, lancing blisters, and attacking other small bodily aberrations.

Slivers

When a piece of wood becomes embedded in your body, either you have been shot with an arrow or you have a sliver. Slivers are usually smaller than arrows, and less painful.

✘ Causes

Touching wood.

☞ Signs and symptoms

1. Slivers are easy to diagnose. Usually, when you get a sliver, you think the chair or the broom has bitten you. This sharp pain is the signal that you have just acquired a sliver.

2. Some slivers are extremely sneaky and sharp, and slip into the skin without calling attention to themselves. If you have a sore spot and you can see something lurking under the skin, this is probably a sliver. The only other thing it could be is a certain kind of parasitical worm common in the Nile River.

The med-tech kitchen

The place to do any kind of surgery, no matter how small, is an operating room. However, you probably don't have an operating room in your house, so you need to adapt one of the other rooms. The kitchen is best. There you have sinks and hot water handy. And chairs and a table, in case you want to have an operating theater.

But if you are to have confidence in the kitchen as an operating room, you will have to outfit it for surgical procedures. You will need equipment that the average French chef has never even heard of. Since other members of

The med-tech kitchen

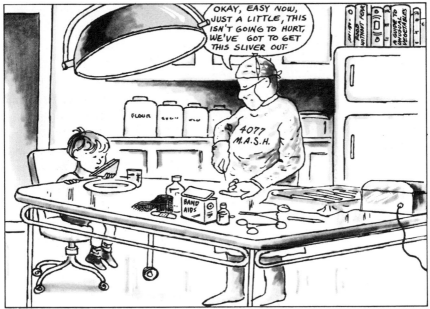

Talk yourself through the operation.

your family may see the kitchen primarily as a place for chopping shallots and eating English muffins, you may find that in properly outfitting it you come into conflict with them.

The solution to this problem lies in the nature of modern medical equipment. It is exquisitely made, and its clean lines and spotless stainless steel fit in well with the prevailing sense of good design. Explain to your family that the successor to hi-tech—the use of industrial materials for home decoration—is med-tech.

You don't have to rush out to a hospital supply store and redo the whole kitchen all at once. Make the changes as you can afford them, and as your family will allow them. These are some of the more important items you might want.

The operating table. A full-sized operating table may seem extravagant, but it makes a dramatic dining room or kitchen table, if you get one that allows you to adjust its height. You don't want to have to eat standing up.

Whatever you do, don't try to disguise the table with a flowery tablecloth. Be bold. Let the

The med-tech kitchen

steel be a statement. And never buy a used table—speculation as to what went on on it may interfere with even your appetite.

The smaller tables used by dog and cat veterinarians are less expensive and make terrific counters. You don't need a cutting board and they are easy to wash.

Lighting. When you go into your own flesh after a sliver you want to be able to see clearly. The dish-shaped reflectors that house lights in operating theaters in hospitals can be adapted for kitchen use with a soft-light bulb. Keep on hand a 10,000-watt bulb for operations.

Silverware. Scalpels make the finest steak knives seem like cudgels. Buy them in quantity. When someone slices through a steak with a scalpel they then realize the ease of living that med-tech brings to the kitchen. Of course, the feeling that you are not cutting a porterhouse, but operating on a cow, turns some people into vegetarians. This simply means less wear and tear on the scalpels.*

Accessories.   Scalpels

*If your family is given to violent arguments over dinner, it is not wise to use scalpels as silverware. They are very sharp.

aren't the only implements that can find new uses in the kitchen. You can use retractor clamps in stuffing a chicken, and sutures to truss it. Surgeon's gloves are good for dishwashing. And surgeon's gowns make great aprons.

Sterilization. The instrument of choice here is an autoclave. In it steam under great pressure is used to sterilize your instruments. Think of it as a dishwasher that gets everything extremely clean. In a pinch it can double as a pressure cooker.

● **Surgical procedure**

1. Don your surgical gown. You need an attendant, or nurse, to help you tie it behind you. Purists leave the gown unadorned. Others have "4077 M*A*S*H" printed on it to add a dash of style.

2. Scrub down with an antibacterial agent. Put on gloves and mask.

3. Put a sewing needle and tweezers in the autoclave. (Scalpels are actually too sharp to use on anything other than dinner. But they do provide the right atmosphere. Have them strewn about the operating table,

The med-tech kitchen

along with retractors and thermometers.)

4. Remove the sewing needle from the autoclave. Gently expose the sliver by pricking up the skin around it and teasing it partly out.

5. Begin to talk yourself through the operation, as if you were instructing medical students in a new procedure. Say things like "Okay, easy now, just a little, this isn't going to hurt, we've got to get this sliver out." Not only will this make you feel like a doctor, it will calm you down if you start to get frightened.

6. Remove the tweezers from the autoclave.

7. Pull out the sliver.

8. Say, "Well now, that wasn't so bad, was it?"

Plague and other horrors

There are certain vicious and deadly diseases that occupy the fringe areas of medical consciousness. Most people assume that these diseases are gone or out of fashion or that you can't catch them in a nice neighborhood. A hypochondriac can't afford to take this kind of cavalier attitude. If you take sickness seriously, you've got to worry about everything. And that includes plague, leprosy, and rabies.

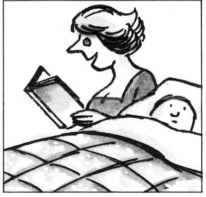

"First the grandma got plague, and then . . ."

Plague

Most people remain unaware of the presence of plague in the United States. But it is here. In the western United States, a variant of bubonic plague hides in the squirrel population the way Nazis still hide in Argentina. If you get bitten by one of these squirrels, you could get plague. In 1981 alone, ten people in the U.S. were stricken with plague.

In any numbers, it is a disease that demands to be taken seriously. The Black Death,

Plague

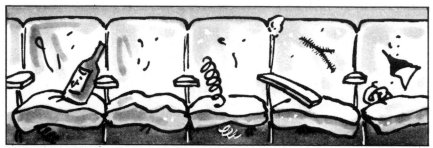

From left: First two seats—sources of plague; next three—sources of leprosy.

which swept through Europe in the fourteenth century, made cancer look like prickly heat. Plague was carried from Asia by rats, and fleas spread the disease from rats to people (beware of anyone who has fleas). The plague killed more than a quarter of the population of Europe. Nowadays, plague stories, told to children at an early age, are one of the causes of hypochondria. All hypochondriacs hold the plague in awe.

It is not likely that we will have a replay of the Black Death. Doctors may be annoying, but they have given us streptomycin. But never mind whether all of Oak Park gets carted off in wagons with torches burning, what about you? What if you happen to be visiting Cody, Wyoming, and you catch bubonic plague from a squirrel? This is a question that cannot fail to concern all hypochondriacs.

☞ Signs and symptoms

1. Swollen glands, listlessness.
2. A high fever.

✖ Sources

1. Rats from Asia.
2. Squirrels from Wyoming.
3. The seats in Times Square movie theaters.

✚ First aid

1. Rest and drink lots of fluids.
2. Call a physician.
3. Call a literary agent. There has not yet been a sentimental, concerned TV movie about someone who gets bubonic plague and is ostracized by friends and family.

Leprosy

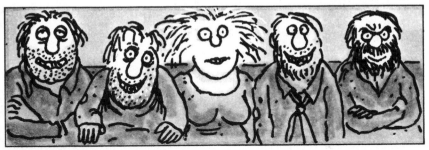

Sources of rabies.

Leprosy

Leprosy is the worst disease you can ever get. It is so bad that the people who have it have tried to change its name to Hansen's Disease to give it a better image.

☞ Signs and symptoms

1. Rashes.
2. Numbness in the fingers and toes.

✗ Sources

1. Lepers.
2. Armadillos. Scientists give armadillos leprosy for experimental purposes. You never know if an armadillo might have escaped from a leprosy lab.
3. The seats in Times Square movie theaters.

✚ First aid

Join a leper colony.

Rabies

Anyone who saw Walt Disney's *Old Yeller* remembers that when the wonderful dog got rabies it turned into a monster, and had to be shot. This movie convinced innumerable young, impressionable hypochondriacs that if Old Yeller could get rabies, no animal could be trusted. Hamsters, gerbils, rabbits, and Pekingese all became suspect members of a great rabid swarm.

Bats also carry rabies. All bats.

☞ Signs and symptoms

1. Excessive salivation.*
2. Uncontrollable excitement.*
3. In the later stages, convulsions.

*This may also be caused by châteaubriand. Make sure you are not in the presence of food.

Rabies

Case history

A young woman was feeding squirrels in a Boston park. She then bought an ice cream cone from a street vendor. After finishing the cone, she became concerned that the squirrel might have had plague. What if, she reasoned, some squirrel saliva had come in contact with her finger? And what if, in the course of eating the cone, she had licked that very same finger? Could she have gotten plague?

She immediately went to a medical student she knew and asked him. The medical student had to call a doctor, since he didn't know the answer. As the potential plague victim listened to the medical student talking on the telephone, she heard him say: "No, she's not crazy. She's usually perfectly sane."

The answer was that not only was it highly unlikely that the squirrel would have had plague (Boston, Massachusetts, is not Cody, Wyoming) but that she would have to have been bitten by the creature. Sharing food with it was not enough. Within a month, the woman had a high fever and swollen glands. Though she recovered, she has never since believed a negative diagnosis.

✗ Sources

1. Foxes and bats.
2. Pet stores.
3. The people in Times Square movie theaters.

✚ First aid

1. Do not shoot yourself.
2. Call a physician—or better yet, a veterinarian.
3. Until help arrives, treat rabies as you would a severe anxiety attack. Rest, undisturbed, in a dark, quiet room. This will prevent convulsions. Also, it can't hurt you if you've made a wrong diagnosis.

Travel sickness

You are planning a vacation, much against your will. Your spouse is looking through travel brochures, reading out loud to you the names of faraway places: India, Ceylon, France. You, on the other hand, are frantically studying a bulletin of the World Health Organization to find out if smallpox really has been eradicated.

For the hypochondriac, every vacation is a terrible adventure. While others merely need to find out where the best restaurants, or ruins, are, you have to find out what you are going to catch. The simple fact that you have to get immunizations before you travel is enough to make you stay home. Why should you go where there is even the remotest chance of getting yellow fever or

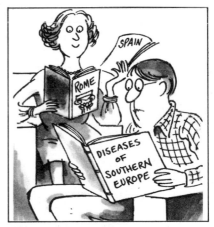

Planning a vacation.

cholera, let alone malaria or sleeping sickness?

Even without these exotic diseases travel is terrifying. You have to be prepared for common illnesses to strike in uncommon circumstances. If there is anything more frightening than having a heart attack, it is having a

Travel sickness

Vacations for the ill

Why look at ruins of temples and risk dysentery when you could have a vacation more suited to your particular interests? Why not a hypochondriac's tour, complete with charter flight and guides? Museums have long been running special tours, led by staff members, for archeology and natural history buffs. Surely, hospitals could do the same for hypochondriacs.

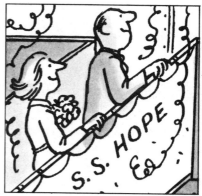

The medical cruise.

The only drawback would be that you would be traveling with a bunch of hypochondriacs. Who would there be to listen to your problems? Still, the tours themselves could be worth it. Some suggestions:

The Hope cruise. A cruise on the medical ship *Hope*. In addition to dancing and dining with some of the world's finest doctors, you receive one free examination and treatment of one medical crisis as part of your fare. (Additional medical attention is extra.) Evening lectures on the world's worst diseases.

Roman pharmacies. See the ruins of the apothecary shops of ancient Rome. Learn what the Romans prescribed for wounds suffered in the arena, and why the Christians were able to tolerate the pain of being eaten by lions. The tour is conducted by a physician fluent in Italian and Latin.

Lourdes holiday. A trip to one of the most famous shrines in the world. Our Lady of Lourdes in France has cured many sick and crippled, whose crutches and headache pills are left at the shrine as signs of their recovery. Sometimes prescribed for hypochondriacs by beleaguered physicians, as in the oft heard "Why don't you go to Lourdes then?"

heart attack in Tirana, the largest city in Albania. Of course, they have socialized medicine, but do they treat capitalists? And how do

Travel sickness

you say, "I'm having a heart attack" in Tosk.*

Similar problems can arise in the most sophisticated of countries. In Paris, for example, sick tourists are not admitted into hospitals unless they have good French accents. The French pretend not to understand what the person is saying.

But, much as you would like to stay home, it will never work. Sooner or later someone is going to pressure you into traveling with them. Inevitably they will pick a place that has crystal waters, great cuisine, and 438 different kinds of intestinal parasites.

If you must travel, bring a letter of introduction from your doctor, and find out the names of the major hospitals you will be near. These additional precautions will also help make your travels more pleasant.

1. Take medicines with you. It is very hard to tell the difference between mouthwash and Liquid Plumber by the Japanese characters on a container.

2. Bring the prescription

*Tosk is the official dialect of Albania. For instructions on what to say if you get sick in Albania, see "Twenty Ways to Say 'I'm Sick.'"

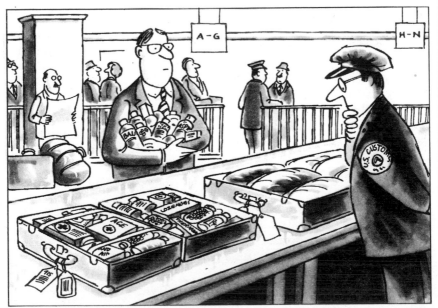

Carry a traveler's medical kit.

In hospital abroad

Before you go traveling, you should know what you are getting into. Some countries are worse than others from a health perspective. Here is a short geographical and statistical* guide.

ALBANIA

POPULATION: 2,730,000
HOSPITAL BEDS (PER 100,000 PEOPLE): 649
PHYSICIANS (PER 100,000 PEOPLE): 104
COMMENTS: Albania is ruled by fanatical communists who believe that although free medical care is a right of the people, diseases are caused by capitalism. Therefore no one is sick. In Albania, hypochondria is considered treason.

CANADA

POPULATION: 23,940,000
HOSPITAL BEDS (PER 100,000 PEOPLE): 875
PHYSICIANS (PER 100,000 PEOPLE): 178
COMMENTS: Canada has the same diseases that the U.S. has, only they are not as severe. This infuriates Canadian nationalists, who are trying to develop some true "Canadian" diseases.

They have not yet been able to do so. The province of Quebec has refused to have anything to do with the rest of Canada and has only French diseases. Instead of headaches, they have *"mal à la tête"*; instead of sore throats they have *"mal à la gorge."*

CHINA

POPULATION: 1,027,000,000
HOSPITAL BEDS (PER 100,000 PEOPLE): 185
PHYSICIANS (PER 100,000 PEOPLE): 33
COMMENTS: If you work—or bathe—in a rice paddy you risk schistosomiasis, a parasitic disease caused by flatworms. The most serious ailment you can contract in China, however, is the cult of personality. An attempt to avoid this malady is the cause of the dull uniformity one sees in China. No one has any personality, on purpose.

FRANCE

POPULATION: 53,710,000
HOSPITAL BEDS (PER 100,000 PEOPLE): 1,125
PHYSICIANS (PER 100,000 PEOPLE): 164

COMMENTS: If you don't speak French fluently, the place will give you a terrible headache. You can also get a bad case of atherosclerosis from the food, and if you are a Francophile, you might contract the ubiquitous "crise de foie"—liver trouble. This is not to be confused with a "crise de foie gras," which is a heart attack brought on by eating large quantities of goose liver pâté.

JAPAN

POPULATION: 116,780,000
HOSPITAL BEDS (PER 100,000 PEOPLE): 1,060
PHYSICIANS (PER 100,000 PEOPLE): 119
COMMENTS: Japan is consensus-oriented, family-oriented, and group-oriented. This means that if anyone in your factory comes down with a cold, so do you. It also means that Japanese hypochondriacs are always thinking other people are sick. The biggest thing to worry about in Japan is raw fish. It tastes delicious, but you can get a tapeworm from it, along with some other odd visitors. Japanese food is also incredibly high in salt, which is bad for high blood pressure. If you are very worried about your diet while visiting Japan, you can stay in Tokyo. The petro-food revolution has hit the Japanese cities and you can always eat fast-food chemical hamburgers.

MONACO

POPULATION: 30,000
COMMENTS: Nobody gets sick in Monaco. It would ruin the country's image.

SWITZERLAND

POPULATION: 6,343,000
HOSPITAL BEDS (PER 100,000 PEOPLE): 1,141
PHYSICIANS (PER 100,000 PEOPLE): 201
COMMENTS: Switzerland is a great place for hypochondriacs to travel. There are no parasites. The whole country is pathologically clean. They have immigration laws to keep out germs and the people the Swiss think carry the germs. There are lots of hospitals and doctors, and they are all incredibly efficient. In fact, the major health problems here are skin ailments brought on by eating too much chocolate.

*Statistics from the *World Almanac and Book of Facts*, 1982.

Malaria

20 ways to say "I'm sick"

ALBANIAN (TOSK): Une jam semur.
ARABIC: Lae ash'or aenni kwaeyyis.*
CHINESE: Wô jué-de bù shū-fu.*
DUTCH: Roep vlug een dokter *(Call a doctor quickly).*
FRENCH: Je suis malade.
GERMAN: Ich bin krank.
GREEK: Eemeh ahrostoss.*
HEBREW: Ani hole.*
ITALIAN: Sono malato.
JAPANESE: Watashi wa byoki desu.*
NORWEGIAN: Jeg er dårlig.
POLISH: Jestem chory/chora *(male/female).*
PORTUGUESE: Estou doente.
RUSSIAN: Yah bolyehn.*
SERBO-CROATIAN: Ja sam bolestan/bolesna/*(male/female).*
SPANISH: Estoy enfermo.
SWAHILI: Ni mogonjwa.
TURKISH: Hastayim.*
YORUBA: ore Ni.
YIDDISH: Eekh vil zikh zen mit ah dawktehr.* *(I wish to see a doctor.)*

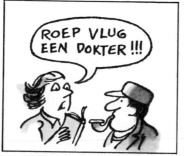

ROEP VLUG EEN DOKTER !!!

*Transliteration from a different alphabet.

slips along with the medicines. This is not for foreign pharmacists, but for customs. One traveling hypochondriac spent three months in a Turkish jail on suspicion of smuggling drugs because of the quantities of pills he was carrying with him. He was finally released because the jailers could not stand the constant complaining.

3. Carry a medical dictionary in the language of the country you are visiting. Regular tourist's phrase books do not give translations for words and phrases like myocardial infarction, CAT scan, and hemorrhoids.

Despite all the precautions, you may still end up with some of the common travelers' ailments.

Malaria

If you go anywhere warm, take protective medication. They say there's no malaria in Florida, but you know there are mosquitoes. Can you trust them?

☞ Signs and symptoms

Fever. If you have a temperature when you're traveling, it's probably malaria.

Motion sickness

✚ First aid

You need rest, and mosquito netting. (You don't want to get bitten again.) See a doctor for drugs as soon as you can.

Be warned, however, that there are now drug-resistant strains of malaria. It might be best not to travel where there are mosquitoes.

Motion sickness

You can't travel without motion, and almost any kind of motion can make you sick. Boats are the worst, but people have been known to become ill from the motion of cars, airplanes, and camels. If you are very sensitive, walking with the wrong gait can make you ill.

Case history

An American on a trip to Paris, armed with old college French, suffered a terrible pain in his chest while walking along the Boulevard St. Michel in the Latin Quarter. He clutched his chest with one hand and raised his other in the air to summon help.

He began shouting in panic, *"Où est l'hôpital?"* One passerby thought he was saying, *"Où est le Pigalle?"* and gave him directions to the red-light district. Fortunately, he couldn't understand them. Other Parisians directed him to the post office, the Ritz, and an outdoor urinal, before he finally found his way to an emergency room.

Once there, and having gained admittance with some difficulty, he found communication with the doctor impossible. Neither had any idea what the other was talking about, so both began speaking more loudly. This did not help. Soon they were shouting at each other. The American left hurriedly when a nurse made him understand that the doctor was trying to decide whether to operate on him for appendicitis or have him arrested for disorderly conduct.

The heart attack turned out to be a false alarm, but the American developed a debilitating fear of French surgeons and had to cut his trip short and go to England.

Montezuma's revenge

Furthermore, the fear of motion sickness all but guarantees that you will get it. This makes motion exceedingly difficult for hypochondriacs, who all know about motion sickness and are all afraid of it.

☞ Signs and symptoms

1. Something similar to food poisoning, without the chills.
2. Despair. Victims of severe motion sickness feel life is not worth living. Tie yourself to the boat, or camel, to prevent yourself from doing something foolish.

✚ First aid

1. If you feel a touch of queasiness, stop all motion. This works for short camel trips. It is harder on planes and boats.
2. For long trips, try to sleep through them. If you can render yourself unconscious before motion sickness strikes, you are safe. You have to be awake to be sick.

Montezuma's revenge

The most famous of traveler's ailments. In fact, travelers can get diarrhea anywhere, simply because the food and water are different. Mexico just happens to have a bad reputation.

☞ Signs and symptoms

1. Loss of weight.
2. Loss of interest in sightseeing.
3. Loss of interest in food.

✚ First aid

1. Don't go sightseeing.
2. Don't eat until you are out of the country.

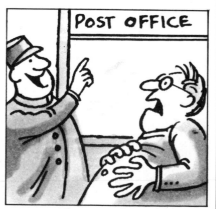

"Non, je suis sick, très sick."

Parasites

Precautions

1. Never eat green meat.

2. Drink only Coca-Cola.

3. Never have the specialty of the house if the house doesn't have indoor plumbing.

Parasites

Anywhere besides Paris, London, and Rome, you are liable to pick up intestinal parasites. After you make any trip, even to Hoboken, have yourself tested. You don't want your stomach to be a lifelong charter flight for unwanted passengers.

Signs and symptoms

1. Loss of weight.

2. Cramps.

3. A feeling that you are not alone.

First aid

Eat the cuisine of a country that is the enemy of the country where you caught the parasites. If you acquired a tapeworm in Syria, drink Israeli wine. If you became sick in Russia, go to a Chinese restaurant. If you catch a parasite in the United States, any country's cuisine will do.

Out of doors

It is unwise ever to venture away from the comforts of medical technology. So you have to think twice about trying to experience the great outdoors. There is the promise of mountain meadows and sweet streams, the beach and the sea. But there are also threats.

The outdoors brings with it a host of new medical dangers—the sun, for example. It has become so widely known that the sun is dangerous that even *Vogue* magazine thinks sunbathing is bad for you (although not as bad as not having a tan). It is plants, not people, that are supposed to lie in the sun. If you can't photosynthesize, you should stay in the shade. In people, direct exposure to the sun causes skin cancer, sunburn, vitamin D poisoning, and a tan. The latter may seem like a good thing, but it has its drawbacks. Nothing hides jaundice like a tan.

Not that this means you should seek out cool weather. The obvious danger there, of course, is freezing to death. More worrisome, because it is insidious, is hypothermia. You can get a fatal case of hypothermia without even getting frostbite.

The other problem with nature is that it is filled with other living things. There are poisonous plants, stinging insects, snakes.* The sad truth is that the primary purpose of all plant and animal life that can't be sautéed in

*Carry a snakbite kit whenever you go where there aren't sidewalks. If a so-called nonpoisonous snake bites you, use your snakebite kit anyway. How can you be sure what kind of snake it is? And who ever saw a snake that didn't look poisonous?

The sun

butter is to afflict human beings. If it won't eat you, bite you, or give you a rash, then it probably carries a disease.

Venture outdoors if you must. But you will soon discover why people invented the indoors.

The sun

If you were lightly toasted all over your body with an acetylene torch, you would turn slightly pink and your skin would hurt. No one would tell you how healthy you look. Nor would you feel refreshed. The sun is just a big torch in the sky and a sunburn is just what it sounds like, a burn.

Unfortunately, in our society, the sun is associated with the beach, and the beach is associated with sex (and diet colas). Consequently, people wear very few clothes at the beach. Scantiness of attire is a tried-and-true method of attracting members of the opposite sex (if you drink diet colas). But in the modern world this only works if you have a tan. Why burned people are thought to be sexy is not known. But millions of Americans in pursuit of sexual adventure also pursue tans. All

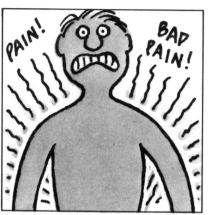

Hypochondriacs don't tan, they burn.

most of them get is sunburned. (They may also get cancer from the diet colas.)

☞ Signs and symptoms

1. Rare. Pink, hot skin, and a desire not to wear clothes that is completely unrelated to sexual drives.
2. Medium. Red skin, great pain, a determination not to let anything or anyone, no matter how attractive they are, touch you anywhere. A desire to die by freezing.
3. Well done. Deep red skin, chills and fever, delirium ending in coma. No desires.

✗ Causes

It is fatuous to blame sun-

The sun

burn on the sun. This is the same twisted logic that blames murders on guns. Here the case is even clearer since "sun control" is impossible. People cause sunburns, usually their own, and usually by lying in the sun too long. Some particularly sad cases get sunburned in tanning parlors under artificial light. Anyone who goes to a tanning parlor deserves to get sunburned.

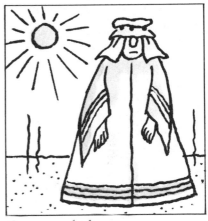

Cover your body.

⇒ **Prevention**

1. Look for love, not sex. Find someone who likes you even if you are fishbelly white. You will be more comfortable, and this is a good sign of a relationship that will last.
2. If you *must* chase the impossible dream, put sun goo on. Use sunscreen, not tanning oil. Hypochondriacs burn, they don't tan. You could always try to ask someone to put the goo on for you. But if you think they might look at your body and make a face, don't risk it. This is the kind of rejection that

brings on severe depression.
3. Beach umbrellas. No one asks people who sit under umbrellas to go to a sex club. This is not all bad. You may attract someone who wants to discuss headaches, or heart disease. Remember, shared interests are more important than gorgeous bodies and great sex.
4. Dress like an Arab. The people of the desert are no fools, they know the sun is their enemy so they cover up every inch of their bodies. (They also practice polygamy.) Not only will this protect you from the sun, people may think you

Hypothermia

are oil-rich and offer to share their bodies with you despite your looks.

✚ First aid

If you insist on trying to be golden brown and beautiful, and fail, take care of yourself in the following ways.

1. For a mild sunburn: Seek out air conditioning. Wear soft clothes. Drink gin and tonics. Admit to yourself that you will never achieve a tan, and that the beach is not for you.

2. For a medium burn: Stay unclothed as much as you can. Pound ice into a fine, snowlike powder and spread it over your body. Keep yourself refrigerated until the pain eases or hypothermia sets in.

3. Well done: Find a hospital with a burn unit. Demand morphine and artificial skin.

Hypothermia

The cold is as dangerous as the sun. It is fairly obvious that you

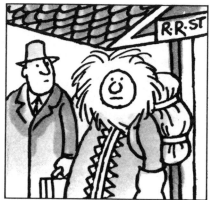

Prevent hypothermia.

can freeze to death, or catch your death of a cold. Less obvious is the insidious threat of hypothermia.

Hypothermia is a slow draining of bodily heat of the sort that occurs when the IRS questions you on the time you took Michael DeBakey to dinner. It is, however, more often the result of actual meteorological cold. Without freezing to death—or even without losing the feeling in your toes—you lose enough heat so that you can become seriously ill and die.

☞ Signs and symptoms

The great danger of hypothermia lies in the silliness of its symptoms, which can trick you into not taking them seriously. Don't make

Hypothermia

that mistake. The symptoms are:

1. Giddiness.
2. Confusion.
3. Stumbling
4. Exhilaration.

These early symptoms are deceptive. At a New Year's Eve party with the windows open, you might experience them all. This presents the truly awesome possibility that you might be seriously ill and yet think you are having a good time. Fortunately, for diagnostic purposes, these ambiguous signs later give way to unmistakable signs of illness:

1. Coma.
2. Death.

✖ Causes

The major cause of hypothermia is hiking in the mountains without proper clothing. But you can get chilled almost anywhere, and there are a number of other situations you should watch out for.

1. Waiting for a bus or commuter train. Last year alone 3,648 commuters in New York, New Jersey, and Connecticut were hospitalized because of hypothermia contracted when their trains were late and they were left to stand in the cold. Food helps prevent hypothermia. If you commute in a cold climate, always carry a knapsack filled with chocolate bars, a small gas stove, and freeze-dried dinners.

2. Air conditioning in movie theaters. If you happen to go to an unpopular movie on an August afternoon, the air conditioning, meant to keep 400 people shivering, can all but freeze you solid. Always carry a heavy sweater to the movies, and the knapsack.

3. Air conditioning in supermarkets. Many a shopper has fallen senseless between the frozen foods and the dairy products. Shop at small grocery stores if you can find them. The prices are higher, but money spent on health is never wasted. If you have to use a supermarket, never go shopping alone—and don't forget your sweater and

Hypothermia

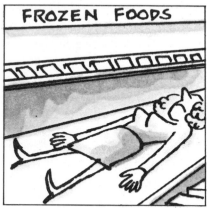

Never shop alone.

knapsack.

4. All winter sports, except bundling. No one who cares about their health plays in the snow. That was the great thing about the discovery of fire. You didn't have to be cold. Now, some people like to be cold because they have been fooled by films of skiing that make it seem that the people are having a good time. Remember, you can't tell from a picture how cold it is.

Bundling, however, is a good winter sport. This is the old practice of getting under a lot of blankets with someone of the opposite sex. It used to be done in haylofts, and both parties would start off fully clothed. Bundling has never been known to cause hypothermia.

✚ First aid

There is a kind of poetic justice to first aid for hypothermia. Since you can think you've got it at almost any time, difficult and unpleasant first aid procedures would be burdensome. One would always be caught between the fear of the illness and the dread of the cure. In hypothermia the cure is always welcome. It is a lot like bundling, and it could happen at the New Year's Eve party even if you didn't know you were ailing.

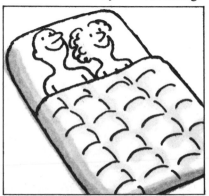

The hypothermia cure.

Plants

1. Take off all your clothes.
2. Have someone else take off all their clothes.
3. Get into a sleeping bag, or under the blankets, together.

Plants

Plants are deceitful. They look harmless. But they are not. Of course, you wouldn't eat a plant that was just growing outside. But you might touch one. And many plants can cause rashes on the skin. Learn to identify poisonous plants. If you know them, you can avoid them.

Poison ivy: Causes an itchy rash if you touch it. Has green leaves, either shiny or dull, smooth or serrated. Usually small, but can be a bush or a vine.

Poison oak: Causes a rash like poison ivy. Has green leaves. Sometimes a shrub, or may look like a tree.

Poison sumac: Causes a very bad rash. Also has green leaves.

☞ Signs and symptoms of poison ivy, oak, and sumac

1. Itching. Terrible, unbearable itching.
2. A red, bumpy rash.

✚ First aid

If you get a poison ivy, oak, or sumac rash:
1. Scratch. Advice not to scratch an incredibly itchy rash is silly. No one could survive. But you don't want to spread the rash or get it on your fingers. Buy a rough towel, one of the old kind used by Puritan

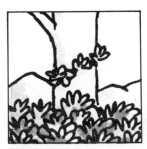

Poison ivy.

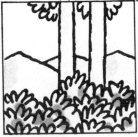

Poison oak.

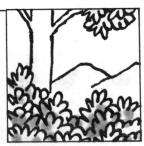

Poison sumac.

Insects

types to stimulate the skin after a cold shower. Cut it into little scratching pads. Rub the affected area with one of these pads with a circular motion, then throw the pad out.

2. "You're gonna need an ocean . . . of calamine lotion." Buy the song "Poison Ivy"; play it over and over. Soon, the song will become so irritating you will forget about your itch.

3. Don't touch anyone else. Above all, don't have sex for the duration of the rash.

Insects

Ecologists contend that all life has a place in a great web. Each organism has its function. The function of insects is to make people miserable, and ill. Not only do bugs sting and bite, they carry diseases. Some insects to avoid, and their diseases:

Bees

Contrary to popular belief, meekness enrages bees. This is even

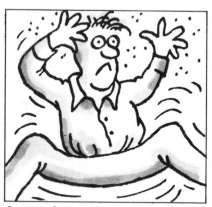
Impress bees with your size and power.

more true for hornets and yellow jackets. If a bee does come near you, don't sit quietly and wait for it to go away like your mother taught you. This will make the bee furious. You are sure to get stung. What you should do is swat at it, scream, run away. Try to get the bee to understand the vast difference in size between you and it, and the power you have to crush its life away, if only you could catch it and hold it without getting stung.

● **Diseases**

Allergic reaction. Bees can kill you if you are allergic to them. And you have to go on the assumption that you *are* allergic to them. Even if you have been stung before and

Insects

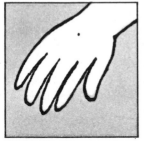

Mosquito bite.

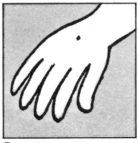

Bee sting.

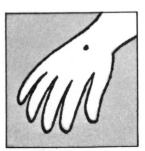

Black fly bite.

didn't suffer extreme swelling and pain, allergies change, and the next time you could find yourself in anaphylactic shock, unable to breathe, the bump swollen to the size of a basketball. Always carry a bee-sting kit, and always use it. Take the pills and give yourself the injection immediately.

Mosquitoes

Mosquitoes, like some hypochondriacs, make a high-pitched whining sound. But only the females bite. Unlike bees, they have no emotional investment in biting humans. They just suck our blood. We are dinner, not enemies. Consequently, nothing you can do in terms of changing your behavior will keep mosquitoes away.

● Diseases

Malaria. Was once prevalent in North America. It could return.

Encephalitis. This inflammation of the brain can cause terrible damage, perhaps resulting in personality disorders and Parkinson's disease. If, after a number of mosquito bites, you find you are unnaturally irritable and shaky, see a doctor.

Ticks

Ticks are very frightening small bugs that attach themselves to animals (including people) and suck blood, which causes the insects to swell up to the size of a pea or larger.

● Diseases

Rocky Mountain spotted fever. Caused by an

Insects

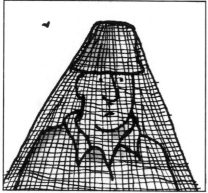

Man against fly.

organism called a rickettsia—something that is halfway between a virus and a bacteria—carried by ticks. As you might expect, the danger is greatest in the Rocky Mountains.
Lyme arthritis. A new disease—the East's answer to Rocky Mountain spotted fever. Discovered near Lyme, Connecticut, this illness is a tick-borne infection that causes an arthritic inflammation. It also afflicts people who wear anything colored lime-green, a color that ticks find obnoxious.

Black flies

These small, biting flies swarm in the spring in northern areas of the North American continent. They leave huge lumps when they bite.

● **Diseases**

Death. Swarms of black flies have been known to kill large mammals. Human beings are large mammals. If you are in black fly country, cover your entire body with fine netting before you go outside.

In the mind

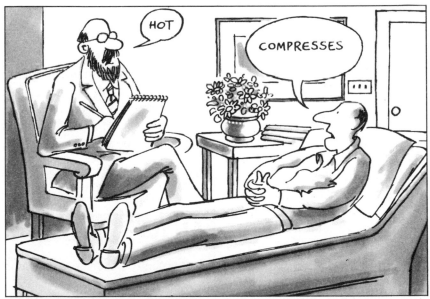

Say whatever comes into your mind.

All hypochondriacs should be in analysis, or traditional psychotherapy—the talking cure. This is not because hypochondria is an illness. Far from it, hypochondria is just a recognition of what life in a world of viruses and chemicals will do to you. You

Depression

may take prickly heat for skin cancer, or a dizzy spell for a stroke. But these are simple mistakes that anyone can make. They don't mean you're crazy.

The reason for analysis is that a hypochondriac does need someone to talk to. And sooner or later friends and family will tire of your symptoms and desert you. All that is left then is to pay someone to listen to you.

The classical Freudians are best, because they hardly ever speak. You, on the other hand, get to say whatever you like. In fact, you are supposed to say whatever you like. If the only things that ever come into your mind are diseases, that is for the analyst to worry about.

Never go to a primal scream, massage, or megavitamin therapist. They won't let you talk. Behavioral therapists will let you get in a word here and there, but they have an awful lot to say themselves. It is a good idea never to pay to hear someone else talk unless he is in a play.

The only drawback to analysis is that, given the hypochondriacal thirst for medical information, you will inevitably read Freud, and dabble in Jung and Adler. This will introduce you to a number of mental illnesses, which you then may think you have. The first thing to do in such a case is to talk to your analyst.

If, for example, you suspect that you are a paranoid schizophrenic, say so. Your doctor will have at his disposal medication for this illness. If he doesn't prescribe medication, you're not a real paranoid. Or, he isn't a real doctor.

You may, however, come down with a mental illness in August, when your psychiatrist is on vacation. Then you will need to try self-diagnosis and first aid. Remember, psychiatrists themselves have trouble figuring out what is wrong with their patients, so don't be discouraged if you can't figure out why you are miserable.

Depression

Depression is the most common mental problem in the United States. In fact, however, depression is usually not an illness at all. There are countless reasons to feel despondent and despairing. Some of them are: nuclear war, inflation, the Mideast, the Mid-

Manic-depressive illness

west. Others are aging, death, punk rock, and "Let's Make a Deal." Why shouldn't you be depressed?

Only when everything in life is going perfectly is depression a sign of mental illness. If you are depressed, try this quick and easy test to tell if you are crazy.

1. Is your job a delight?
2. Are you lucky in love?
3. Do you have enough money?

If you answered yes to all three questions, something is seriously wrong with you whether or not you are depressed. If you answered no to any of them, you have every reason to be depressed.

☞ Signs and symptoms

1. Unhappiness
2. Lack of interest in chocolate.
3. Severe lethargy, similar to symptoms of leukemia.

✚ First aid

1. Whistle a happy tune.
2. Eat. Anything.
3. Make a lot of appointments for leukemia tests; it

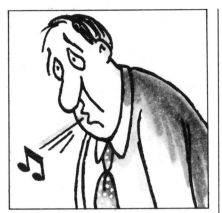

Whistle a happy tune.

will give you something to think about and take your mind off the depression.

Manic-depressive illness

While depression is nothing to worry about, mania is something else. Periods of energetic happiness, approaching exhilaration, are not normal. They make your usual, everyday unhappiness seem like clinical depression. And exhilaration can be dangerous for someone in generally ill health. If you find yourself overjoyed, you should suspect mental illness.

Schizophrenia

Signs and symptoms

1. Excess happiness.
2. Lack of interest in illness.
3. Overwhelming optimism.

✚ First aid

The most important thing here is not to let the illness become chronic. You don't want to end up as one of those people who chatter and sing at breakfast. Read medical journals. This will bring you down to earth.

Schizophrenia

Schizophrenia is the cancer of mental illness. Schizophrenics are completely out of touch with reality and often have no sense of what language means or how to wear their hair. Often their thoughts are very odd.

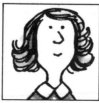

Normal hair.

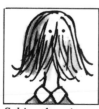

Schizophrenic hair.

Schizophrenia usually strikes the young, probably because older people are too depressed to have such a demanding illness.

☞ Signs and symptoms

1. A belief that you are a world leader or religious prophet.
2. Poor taste in clothes. This does not mean wearing your skirts too long, but rather wrapping your head in newspapers and plastic bags and using large cardboard boxes for shoes.
3. You have conversations with inanimate objects.
4. Inanimate objects have conversations with you.

✚ First aid

1. Find out if other people think you are a world leader or religious prophet. After all, Napoleon thought he was Napoleon too.
2. Don't talk to anything you haven't seen a sane person talk to. For instance, everyone talks to red lights. But nobody talks to curbs. If they talk to you, don't listen.
3. Bathe. The importance

Split personality

of personal hygiene cannot be overestimated. People are willing to overlook extraordinary aberrations in behavior if you wash often and have sweet breath.

4. If you are very worried that you have caught schizophrenia, and your psychiatrist is away, make a list of facts about your life that suggest that you are just like everyone else; put down your job, your friends, your girlfriend, your hobbies, your happy moments. This should get you through August.

5. If you have no job, no friends, no girlfriend, no hobbies, and no happy moments, you are safe in believing that you have a serious problem. This is not something that a shave and a haircut can take care of. Find out who your psychiatrist left to care for his patients while he's away and make a quick appointment.

Split personality

You may wonder, at times, what possessed you to eat that carcinogenic hot dog, or to go to work when you had sneezed that morning. What made you tell the doctor you felt fine? Of course, you may be tempted to brush these incidents off with a simple "Oh, I wasn't myself this morning." But you should stop to think in such a situation, and ask yourself, "Well then, who was I?"

☞ Signs and symptoms

1. Do you find empty milk cartons in the refrigerator, and wonder who put them there?

2. Does your laundry come back with socks that you don't recognize?

3. Do strangers call you on the telephone asking for

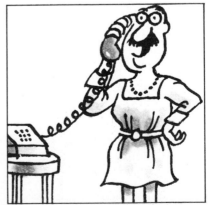

"There's no Estelle here. Or is there?"

Hypochondria

Free association by hypochondriac

WORD	ASSOCIATION
lung	*cancer*
liver	*cancer*
stomach	*cancer*
heart	*disease*
cold	*sore*
hot	*compresses*
sexual	*dysfunction*
doctor	*bills*
swine	*flu*
broken	*leg*
hay	*fever*
sick	*yes*
well	*no*
good	*diagnosis*

people you have never heard of?

4. Do you wake up with tattoos you don't remember getting?

✚ First aid

1. Set traps for your other selves. Put salt in the milk and see if you drink it. Leave a tape recorder on all night.

2. Look out for traps set by your other selves for you. Is there salt in the milk? Was the tape recorder left on all night?

3. See a dermatologist about the tattoos.

4. Relax, and enjoy the company. Everyone loves to hear about split personalities, so you will be very popular. And you won't have to go far to find a date.

Hypochondriac's hypochondriac

This is a truly severe psychological syndrome, in which the victim, who is perfectly healthy and never talks about feeling sick, thinks he is a hypochondriac, and is constantly complaining about it. There is no cure.

The Hippocratic curse

You can't take care of everything with first aid. Sooner or later you will have to see a doctor; probably more than one. And this is likely to cause a tumult of contradictory emotions.

On the one hand, it is a great thing to be talking to someone who also has illness as his major interest in life, particularly someone who has been to medical school. Stethoscopes, white coats, and illegible handwriting all inspire a feeling of awe. And nothing can compare with the feeling of gratitude and relief when a doctor tells you the bumps on your arm are not skin cancer, but warts.

On the other hand, it is upsetting to have the doctor contradict your own diagnosis. And nothing is worse than getting one of those doctors who won't listen, won't talk to you, and doesn't seem to know what he is doing. Even if the doctor seems to be a good one, stethoscopes and tongue depressors lose their aura of importance the farther you get from the doctor's office. On your way home, inevitably, you begin to wonder just where he went to medical school. Naples, Bogotá, Teheran? How do you know he was right about the warts?

For a hypochondriac, however, there is no way around doctors; they are absolutely necessary. Without them there would be no prescriptions, no X-rays, no physical examinations—no illness as we know it. So you have to put up with a lot from them, but not everything. When you call to find out the results of your blood test,

Finding a doctor

and the doctor tells you that your collarbone is broken, it is time to find a new physician.* You may never find one who sticks to his appointment schedule, but you ought to be able to get one who remembers who you are.

In order to get along with doctors you need to learn certain special skills, the first of which is how to find a good one.

Finding a doctor

If you have a doctor, and you need a specialist, you can ask your own doctor to refer you to one. If you have a bad doctor and you want to find a good one, this is more difficult. There are different ways to find doctors.

1. Friends. Only ask friends who are hypochondriacs. A health chauvinist (if you associate with that sort of person) is liable to send you to a doctor who thinks that anything short of a broken limb will "take care of itself."

Tell your friends that you are looking for these qualities in a doctor:

(a) Reads your file before he talks to you.

(b) Talks to you, rather than making rhetorical first person plural pronouncements, as in "Well, we're sick today, are we?"

(c) Sticks to the subject at hand. Nothing is worse than a chatterbox proctologist who says things like "How about those Dodgers?" during examinations.

2. Medical journals. Go to the library and do some research on your health problem. If a doctor in your area has published a research paper on it, see him. You might even find a new illness in perusing the journals, as well as a doctor. However, you should never tell a doctor that you read medical journals. They don't like the competition.

3. The emergency room. You may meet a doctor you like on one of your visits to the emergency room.

The waiting room

When you have found a doctor, made an appointment, and reached the waiting room, you may think that this is half the

*And to get your collarbone X-rayed.

The waiting room

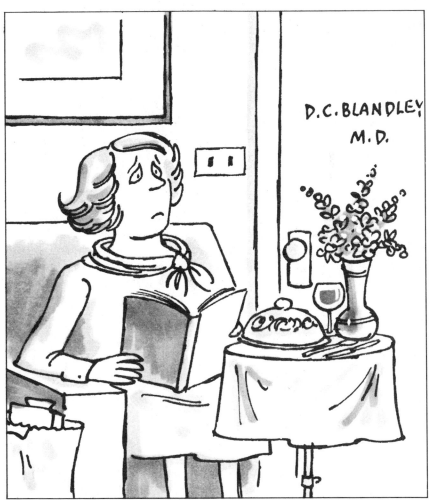

Always bring a snack to the waiting room.

battle. It is not; it is the beginning of the battle. Some people who have spent much of their life in waiting rooms believe that doctors make their patients wait one half hour or an hour because they want to torture them. Others, of a more generous nature, think that although doctors may be medically skilled, both they and the people they hire to keep their appointments straight are com-

Doctor's horoscope

It is helpful to know the personality traits of the doctors you deal with. Some people think the stars determine personality. They judge what a person is like by how the stars and planets were arranged on the person's birthdate. Most doctors won't tell you when they were born, but there is another method you can use. Doctors are sorted out during medical school according to their personalities, and assigned to certain specialties. Each specialty has its own personality type. Examples:

wish they had been cardiologists.

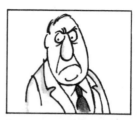

Proctologist. An unhappy group, and understandably so. Spending your life looking for hemorrhoids and cancer of the colon is enough to make anyone sour and grim. They wish they had been internists.

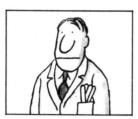

Internist. The internist has replaced the old general practitioner, or family doctor. Internists are among the friendliest of doctors, although they are often bland and unexciting. They constantly deal with the same boring old stomach problems and checkups, and they never get any medical glory. They are often round-shouldered. They

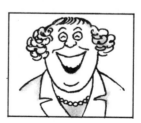

Gynecologist. Male gynecologists are distressingly cheerful; female gynecologists disturbingly serious. The choice is often between one who calls you "dear" and thinks of his patients as "girls," and one who hums "Solidarity Forever" as she examines you. Gynecologists, like proctologists, act bored by their work, but the gynecologists are faking it.

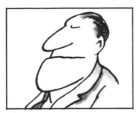

Brain surgeon. They consider themselves the test pilots of the medical world; they have the "right stuff." They drive fast cars, are arrogant, and push people around. This is okay. You wouldn't want to play tennis with a brain surgeon, but when you're shopping for a doctor to cut into your head, you want one who is sure of himself.

Psychiatrist. No one knows what they are like, since they never talk.

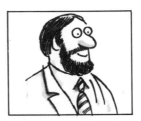

Young country doctor. He is never silent, insists on telling you in great detail what he is doing and why, since he believes in patients' rights. He thinks there is nothing wrong with marijuana, if you grow it yourself so that it is not contaminated with herbicides. He is also interested in sports medicine and believes there may be something to holistic healing. Doesn't shave on purpose.

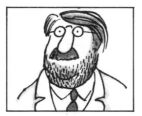

Old country doctor. He is usually silent, old, and doesn't believe there is anything wrong with cholesterol, or bourbon. He will never tell you what the medication he prescribes is. Whether he is giving you a shot or pills, all he says is, "This ought to fix you up." Sometimes forgets to shave.

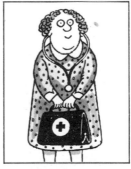

Mom. Small, gray-haired, particularly adept at stomachaches and poison ivy. Specialty is pediatrics, but she is often useful for a second opinion no matter how old you are. Makes house calls.

Doctor-patient etiquette

pletely and utterly incompetent at organizing a schedule.

Neither of these beliefs is true. The actual explanation has to do with a little-known branch of mathematics that is a required course in all medical schools. The course is called Telling Time. The first principle of telling time for doctors is:

1. Time is money.

The second is that there are two kinds of time, each worth different amounts of money— Doctor's Time and Patient's Time. The different kinds of time are worth:

1. Doctor's Time—$200 an hour or more.

2. Patient's Time—nothing.

Consequently, you must be prepared for a long wait. Always arrive 15 minutes late yourself. Plan to delay paying your bill one month for each extra 15 minutes you have to wait. Other rules:

1. Bring a snack.

2. Bring your own reading material. Doctors have terrible taste in magazines.

3. If you have to wait a long time, you can encourage the doctor to see you sooner by:

(a) Asking frequently what the problem is that is causing the delay. Pretend you don't know that such waits are common.

(b) Asking to use the phone. Call someone and talk loudly about how long you have been waiting. If everyone in the waiting room turns to look at you, you are talking loudly enough.

(c) Moaning in pain.

(d) Fainting.

Doctor-patient etiquette

Doctors are very busy, very impatient people. If you are to get anything out of your meeting with the doctor, write out everything you want to say beforehand. Otherwise, in the heat of the moment, when he is taking your medical

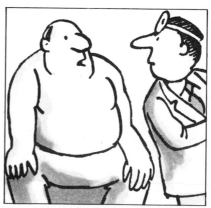

"Do you think I'm an ectomorph?"

Doctor-patient etiquette

Case history

A middle-aged man, on a hike, twisted his ankle, aggravating an earlier injury to the same ankle. He managed to finish the hike, despite the pain, because he was trying to hide his hypochondria from his fellow hikers. After several days of hobbling around, the ankle still pained him, and it had started to show some ominous colors.

He went to the emergency room where, much to his shame, he was fobbed off on a physician's assistant. However, X-rays were taken, and they seemed to show a chip fracture. An orthopedic surgeon had to be called in for a second opinion. Two nurses arrived to get in on what was shaping up to be an interesting case. The man's spirits were picking up.

When the surgeon arrived he poked at the man's ankle and asked a few questions, then announced that the apparent chip must have been either an old injury or a deformity in the bone, since it was nowhere near the location of the pain. Faces fell all around. The physician's assistant and the two nurses immediately lost interest in the patient. The surgeon left without saying good-bye. The man was sent home in medical disrepute with an Ace bandage and a bill.

Within a few days, the ankle was better, and the man had recovered from his embarrassment. He had also begun to think about those X-rays. What about that bone chip? What was he doing with a deformed ankle? Could that be what was causing his backaches? He decided to make an appointment with another orthopedic man. No point in letting a good set of X-rays go to waste.

history, you may forget that your father had eczema.

It is particularly important to write down all your symptoms, including times and intensity of the particular symptom. For this reason it may be appropriate to keep a medical diary.

In order to find out what is wrong with you, you must be quick and persistent. Otherwise, many doctors will just say things are fine, or give you a prescription and mumble something and send you on your way. In order to get information out of a reticent

The emergency room

doctor you must ask very specific questions.

If you ask how your EKG turned out, the doctor will probably say, "Everything is normal." This is not what you want to hear. Ask instead something like "Do I have premature ventricular contractions?" A question like that always wakes a doctor up. He'll probably respond in much more detail. Other good questions are:

"Do you think I'm an ecto-morph?"

"What about the triglyc-erides?"

"Could it be diverticulitis?"

"Is this a placebo?"

You may also run into one of those doctors who think that having an M.D. is like being a feudal lord. Veterinarians are nicer to heifers than these doctors are to you. Even though your natural reverence for the medical profession may make it difficult, you have to take strong action in such cases.

If the doctor is very unpleasant, don't have him bill you, and don't give a check to his secretary. Pay him in cash, and tip him. Say, "I would have given you more if your hands weren't so cold." Doctors hate this. They

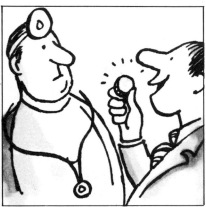

"This is for you."

never like to be reminded of where their money comes from.

The emergency room

As a hypochondriac you will find that emergency rooms are a kind of home away from home. When the midnight heart attack gets out of hand, when appendicitis strikes yet again, there is no other recourse.

After a few visits, however, it will become apparent that the only good thing about emergency rooms is that they are open 24 hours a day. The rest is awful. For one thing, the waiting room is usually filled with sick and injured people. This will make you

The emergency room

feel that your own complaint is not good enough, and you will be tempted to leave. Don't. You might actually have appendicitis this time. You have to learn not to doubt yourself. You don't have to have a gunshot wound to go to the emergency room. You just have to have an "emergency." One of the principles of hypochondria is that every human being has a different emergency threshold. For some, bleeding or incapacitating pain is necessary. For others, the fear of blood or pain is quite enough.

If you have exhausted first aid measures (and your family), and your doctor is not available, don't hesitate. That's what the emergency room is there for.

● **Emergency room protocol**

1. When you describe your complaint to the nurse, don't act sheepish. Just state straightforwardly what you feel and what you think your problem is. Emergency room personnel are used to people coming in at 3:00 A.M. with canker sores. All they want to do is write up your form as quickly as possible and

Medical diary

December 21

8:00 A.M. The start of winter. Here comes the flu, and I've just gotten over that cold. Woke up this morning with tightness in the chest. Bronchitis? Remember to tell Dr. Barnes about the pleurisy when I see him.

10:00 A.M. Just remembered I haven't bought Aunt Lillith her gift. Nauseated.

Lunch. Intense chest pains, heart skipped beat during lunch with boss. Tried not to show it, but it was hard to talk and take pulse at the same time. Did he notice? Remember to tell Dr. Friedman about the arrhythmia.

3:00 P.M. Foot hurts. Arthritis? Tell Dr. Balthazar.

8:00 P.M. Started wrapping gifts. Felt sick. Awful taste in mouth. Must be an ulcer, unless it's those stickers I've been licking. Have to ask Dr. Kennedy if there are neurotoxins in the glue on Christmas stickers.

4:00 A.M. Can't decide if this should be tomorrow's entry. Woke up with big fear of death. Had dream that heart stopped in doctor's office, but couldn't remember which doctor it was and they wouldn't let me see him until I guessed his name right. Had to wait three hours with heart not beating. When I saw the doctor he said it was nothing. Maybe I need a new cardiologist.

The emergency room

find out what insurance you have.

2. There will always be at least one person waiting who has had a psychotic breakdown. Do not look at him. Even if he shouts at you or makes comments about your socks, don't look at him. Mental illness can be transmitted by eye contact.

3. Do not offer to give up your place in the waiting order for someone who looks worse off. Broken ankles can wait. If the nurses think someone is seriously injured, they'll put him first. Nobility and hypochondria don't mix.

4. When you do get to see the doctor, don't try to pretend you are not terrified. Trying to impress a doctor with bravery always backfires. If you are so brave, he will reason, you shouldn't be in the emergency room with canker sores. The doctor will only be irritated at you for taking up his time. But if he sees that you are truly in fear for your life, that you think the sores may be a sign of lymphatic cancer, he will be more thorough in examining you and more pleasant in explaining to you how to gargle with salt water. Be sure to thank him profusely and show enormous relief. Doctors like this, particularly those who are stuck in the emergency room, where many of their patients are unconscious.

5. Finally, don't go to the same emergency room twice in one month. Repeat visitors are often not taken seriously.

Home health care

Nutrition

Food is widely recognized to be essential to life. Unfortunately, scientists have recently discovered that it is also a major cause of death. This makes it hard to figure out what to eat.

Food gives you heart disease, high blood pressure, and cancer. It can also make you crazy. You can become an anorexic, or a bulimic. Food is also filled with deadly "calories," which cause obesity and other ailments. Even the best food, if you eat too much of it, will kill you.

Death and disease lurk on every side. Suppose you're cutting down on fats and you decide to go vegetarian. Then you forget to combine the right foods to get the right proteins and before you know it you've got kwashiorkor,

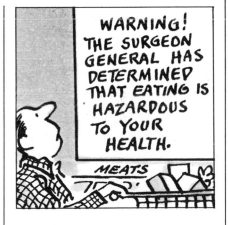

a protein deficiency disease. Or, even worse, as a vegan (a person who eats no animal products, not an alien on "Star Trek") you forget to take your vitamin B_{12} tablets and you end up with nerve damage and megaloblastic anemia. Having a disease like that, plus never getting to eat steak or ice

Principles of nutrition

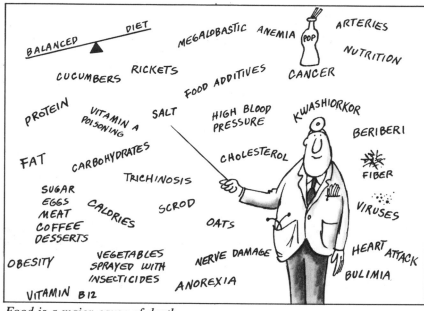

Food is a major cause of death.

cream, is too much.

Still, special diets do have their compensations. For example, you may have decided that you have high blood pressure, despite what the doctors say. So you eliminate salt from your diet. This may sound like a terrible burden, but you can ease it by serving the same diet to your guests. Nothing turns the conversation around to high blood pressure like a no-salt cracker. And what could be a better topic of conversation for a dinner party?

● Basic principles of nutrition:

1. Eat less than seems possible. Modern nutritional experts believe it is healthful to be hungry all the time. If you feel satisfied and content after a meal, you have eaten too much.

2. Never eat anything that tastes good. Scientists have discovered that all the things that taste good—sugar, salt, porterhouse steak, cheesecake—are haz-

Cholesterol fiber

ardous to your health.
3. Eat poor. Imagine that you are either a peasant or a hunter-gatherer, and eat accordingly. Nuts, berries, and brown rice will keep you healthy.
4. Eat a balanced diet. This means that you should have lots of different nuts and berries.

High in cholesterol
Prime rib
Lobster
Butter
Whipped cream

Low in cholesterol
Scrod
Lettuce
Wax beans
Jerusalem artichokes

Cholesterol

Certain substances in food are tremendously dangerous, and cholesterol is one of them. Cholesterol is the chemical that ruined meat's reputation. Although it is a substance that the body needs, it also tends to cause a buildup of "plaque" on the interior walls of arteries. It is as if the Lincoln Tunnel got narrower every time certain kinds of cars drove through it. One day, the cholesterol blobules clog the whole thing up, causing a major heart attack.

Cholesterol is present in most good food. In fact, a sure way to tell whether you should eat something if you are cutting down on cholesterol is to taste it. If you like it, it has cholesterol.

Fiber

Doctors have recently come to believe that food with no nutritional value whatsoever is good for you. Fiber is food that you can't digest. It used to be called roughage. Being indigestible and otherwise useless, it passes through the intestinal system quickly, scouring out the plumbing and keeping it in good working order.

Foods with fiber
Bran
Oats
Hay
Wood chips

Foods with no fiber
Crème caramel
Milk shakes
Filet mignon
Chocolate

Vitamins

Vitamins

Certain segments of the health food community feel that vitamins have religious significance. You may be offered a vitamin with a glass of wine, or by itself, in the middle of the day. The act always has a sacramental feeling to it, and Roman Catholic hypochondriacs may be tempted to mumble some Latin as they receive the tablet of vitamin C.

Actually, doctors say that big doses of most vitamins don't do much good. Some vitamins can even poison you. But it is true that lack of certain vitamins causes horrible diseases, which every hypochondriac should know about.

Here are some of the more important vitamins, their deficiency diseases and their reputed effects.

Vitamin A

If you can't see in the dark, you have a vitamin A deficiency, which also causes retarded growth. Fortunately, vitamin A is present in fruits, vegetables and dairy products. Unless you are eating a diet of sand and gravel (mega-macrobiotic), you will probably get enough of it. How-

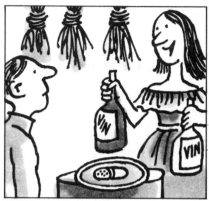

"White with the B-complex?"

ever, excess vitamin A is poisonous, so you may want to limit your consumption of fruits, vegetables, and dairy products.

Vitamin B₁ (Thiamine)

Deficiency causes beriberi. It is present in liver, whole grains, yeast, and nuts. Or, if you are willing to risk trichinosis, you can get it in pork.

Vitamin C

The king of vitamins. Lack of it causes the famed scurvy. A lot of it, it is now claimed, will prevent colds and cure cancer. For these effects, you must take it in very large doses. If the pill is difficult for you to swallow because of its size, the dose is probably large enough. If you are serious about vitamin C, you can get chewable tablets and eat them like candy all day long.

Vitamins

A day in the diet

A sample menu for an average day, with the effects of the foods you normally eat.

Breakfast

Two eggs, bacon, toast with butter, and coffee.

Effects: Cholesterol in eggs and bacon and butter on toast causes atherosclerosis; nitrates in bacon cause cancer; coffee increases your risk of cancer of the pancreas; caffeine in coffee causes caffeine addiction with resulting headaches, anxiety, and other symptoms.

Lunch

Pastrami on rye, potato chips, pickles, cola, and cheesecake for dessert.

Effects: Everything in this lunch comes under the heading of "Death Food." It all tastes great, but its nutritional value is totally outweighed by its evil effects on the body. The pastrami is heavy with fat and chemicals—heart disease and cancer; the potato chips and pickles have enormous amounts of salt—high blood pressure; the cola is composed entirely of sugar and petrochemicals—it will upset your body's metabolism and corrode your esophagus; cheesecake enters the arteries whole and can cause heart attacks and sudden obesity. The ambulance may have to come directly to the delicatessen.

Dinner

Japanese pickled vegetables, assorted sushi, tempura, sake.

Effects: At first glance this may seem to be an admirable meal. However, Japanese pickled vegetables are pure salt, the sushi carries fish tapeworm and other parasites, the tempura is fried in oil, and new evidence shows that although polyunsaturated oil is good for the heart, it may cause cancer. The sake will give you a terrible hangover.

Vitamin D

Lack of this substance will cause rickets, which supposedly occurs only in children. If you see that you are bowlegged, however, you might want to eat a lot of egg

Additives

yolks, milk, and fish oil. Of course, you have to weigh the risk of rickets against the dangers of cholesterol. Another solution is to lie in the sun, which helps the body make its own vitamin D. This causes skin cancer.

Additives

Food is not just food. There are a lot of other things in it—preservatives, dyes, artificial flavorings, and colorings. All of them cause cancer.

➡ **To avoid getting cancer from food:**

1. Read the label. If there is any ingredient you can't pronounce, this is not something you should buy.

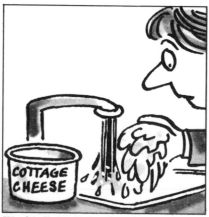

Wash all fresh food.

2. Beware of pesticides and other chemicals. Wash all fresh food thoroughly. This includes butter and cottage cheese.
3. Never eat or drink anything that will clean a copper penny.

The ethics of food

What you eat is a matter of moral as well as medical concern. And as a hypochondriac you may want to stop and give thought to your spiritual well-being, particularly since food morality is supposed to coincide with health. Many people have stopped eating meat altogether, because they believe it is not only unhealthful but immoral to kill and eat cows and chickens.

They are probably right. Of course, you may say you are not in good enough health to worry about saving other human beings, let alone chickens. This argument infuriates ethical vegetarians, who say that human beings are in no way morally more valuable than chickens. Again, they are probably right. But there is also a question as to whether human be-

The ethics of food

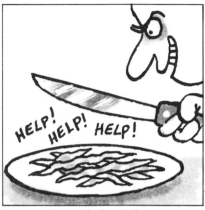

Do wax beans feel pain?

ings are morally more valuable than wax beans. For most human beings (and most wax beans) the answer is no. This sends you back to the sand-and-gravel diet.

You may choose to stop eating meat, but you should know that you will have to spend the rest of your life trying to figure out whether you have the right combination of proteins in your vegetarian diet. This will cause you to end up eating huge numbers of beans.

If you decide to go vegetarian, these will be the sorts of things you will eat:

Bulgur
Brown rice
Kidney beans
Red beans
String beans
White beans
Wax beans
Kasha
Kohlrabi
Carrots
Spinach
Cabbage
Seaweed

If you don't become a vegetarian, these will be the sorts of things you will eat:

Saltimbocca à la Romana
Filet mignon with sauce béarnaise
Barbecued ribs
Turkey with stuffing
Steak tartare
Roast pork with gravy

Make your own decision.

Exercise

Hypochondriacs would like to exercise. It is now known that unless you run a marathon you will die of a heart attack. But, as a hypochondriac, you also know that you can die of a heart attack during a marathon.

This is a modern dilemma. Hypochondriacs 20 years ago did not have to exercise. Then, being still was a good way to avoid having a heart attack. People only ran if they were being chased. Now you are supposed to get all sweaty and make your heart beat fast in order to make it healthy, an idea that seems to go against nature.

Nonetheless, almost all doctors now say that exercise is good for you. If you don't exercise, you will feel terribly guilty, and socially isolated. But you can't just put on sneakers and run around the block. What if your heart has a hidden defect? First, get a stress electrocardiogram. If you collapse during this test, at least there will be a lot of doctors and defibrillators around.

If you live through your stress test, then you may choose a form of exercise. But be careful. Weigh the ailments that result from doing the exercise against those that result from no exercise. It is all a matter of risks and benefits. If you jog you keep your heart and lungs in good working order. But while your heart thrives, your feet may not. Having a strong heart is small compensation if you are unable to walk.

Exercise also puts you in touch with your body, since you

Muscular fitness

have to monitor your pulse with extra care and pay attention to stretching your muscles and maintaining your ligaments. For a health chauvinist this is probably good, since it helps him know when he has broken a bone. You, on the other hand, have no doubt already established a lively dialogue with your body. Fostering a heightened awareness of the body in a hypochondriac is something like putting Vlad the Impaler in touch with his anger. The results can be frightening.

To limit the hazards of exercise and make it more appropriate for someone in your state of health, follow these basic principles.

● Basic principles of exercise

1. Never exercise alone. If you jog, jog with a group so there will be someone to run for help if you collapse on the track. If you don't have any friends, have an ambulance follow you.
2. Less is enough. If you are following an exercise plan keyed to age, use the plan for people ten years older than you are.
3. During every exercise,

take your pulse.
4. After every exercise, check yourself for injuries.

Muscular fitness

Exercises for muscular fitness can make you strong, or flexible, or beautiful. You can end up looking like Baryshnikov, or Jane Fonda. Of course, if you overdo it you could also end up looking like Arnold Schwarzenegger. But overdoing exercise is not a problem for hypochondriacs.

But is muscular fitness good for your health? Well, yes and no. Poor muscular fitness causes backaches, slipped discs, pinched nerves, and innumerable aches and pains. Unfortunately, doing the exercises to improve muscular fitness can also cause backaches, slipped discs, pinched nerves, and innumerable aches and pains.

If you don't do the exercises you will both hurt and look flabby and ugly. If you do the exercises you will still hurt, but you will look a little bit better (don't hope for too much). This is good because people are always more willing to sympathize with an attractive hypochondriac.

Old-fashioned muscle fit-

Muscular fitness

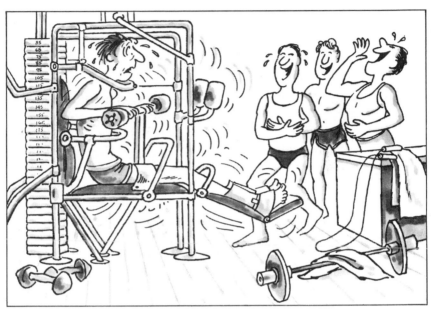

With exercise machines, you run the risk of being trapped.

ness exercises include standards such as push-ups and sit-ups. You can do these in the privacy of your own home. For some reason, no one does this anymore, perhaps because it feels so tawdry to be sweating on the living room floor. Nowadays, people join health clubs so that they can sweat in front of a mirror.

The new machines

The current proliferation of health clubs has brought to the public exotic muscle training machines made of chrome and leather. These machines, based on recently discovered drawings by the Marquis de Sade, are set in mirrored rooms with plush carpets. The health clubs hire people who have already achieved cosmetically obvious muscular fitness to parade around with few clothes on and instruct novices in the mysteries of the new machines.

Because of the machines and the bodies of the instructors, the novice feels that he is involved in a highly serious form of exercise, if not a major sexual perversion. This is very different

Aerobic exercise

from doing sit-ups on plastic-covered mats at the YMCA.

- ## Benefits of machine exercise

1. If you use the machines correctly, you will gain a feeling of vigor, a better-looking body, and a new willingness to go to the beach.
2. Even if you only fool around, you still get to watch other people watch themselves in the mirror, a complicated form of voyeurism.

- ## Disadvantages of machine exercise

1. Infection. The machines, on which many people sweat, are ideal breeding grounds for bacterial and fungus infections. A strong back is not much good if it is covered with green rot.
2. Entrapment. There is always the possibility that one of the machines will close up its chrome and leather limbs on you and refuse to let you out. This makes the insecure and flabby afraid that all the people who have already achieved muscular fitness will laugh at them for being too weak to get out of the machine.

- ## Muscular fitness for the ill

1. Never use a machine that has a neck strap.
2. If you can't make the machine move at all, ask if they have one with a motor.

Aerobic exercise

The heart and lungs make up the cardiovascular system. It is responsible for getting oxygen into the body, and then sending it out to the muscles in the blood.

Certain kinds of exercise improve the functioning of the cardiovascular system. They are called aerobic exercises, and it is easy to tell which ones they are. If an exercise makes you feel out of breath, it is aerobic.

Jogging

This is now the most common form of exercise in the country. The reason for this is that it is not hard to learn. Enormously uncoordinated people can learn to jog

Jogging

in a matter of weeks. Consequently, previous humiliating experiences in junior high gym classes should not keep you from jogging.

● Benefits

1. Helps you breathe.*
This cuts down the risk of heart attacks.
2. Makes it easier to catch buses. And, if you don't catch the bus, not to worry, you can always jog to work.

● Disadvantages

1. Musculoskeletal havoc.

Constantly pounding the pavement ruins your feet, knees, hips, back, and neck. Joggers are usually in pain. They don't smile and are not happy people. But you won't want to associate with other joggers because they tend to monopolize the complaining.
2. Makes your calf muscles look stringy.

● Jogging for the ill

1. Don't try to go fast.

*This is true of all aerobic exercises.

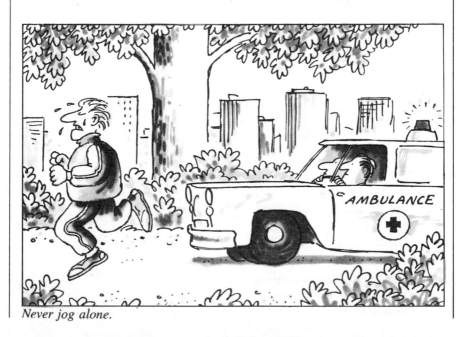

Never jog alone.

Bicycling/Aerobic dance

That is running. You don't ever want to run. Jogging is not much faster than walking, just bouncier.
2. Don't set your goals too high. Let other people measure their jogging in miles. Measure yours in yards.
3. Unless you have an electronic pulse monitor, don't swing your arms while you jog. You need to be able to take your pulse all the time. Watch for danger signs. A heavy "thump" heartbeat, or anything over 90 beats a minute, should warn you to stop.

Bicycling

Bicycling is an alternative to jogging. It is a lot easier on the skeleton, but requires more coordination than jogging.

● Benefits

1. Not only do you get healthy, you go fast. Bicycling is actually a form of transportation, as opposed to jogging, during which most people run around in circles.

2. The wear and tear is not on your knees and feet, but on the bicycle.

● Disadvantages

1. To deal with the damage done to the bicycle you go to a bicycle mechanic, not a doctor. You cannot talk to a bicycle mechanic about pains in your chest.
2. You have to wear silly hats and tight black shorts.
3. You have to compete with automobiles. While joggers can hide in parks or run on tracks, bicyclists are right out there on the streets. Jogging injuries are bearable. Being run over by a car is not.

● Bicycling for the ill

1. Use a three-speed. That will be more than enough for you to handle. You won't need the extra gears because you should never bicycle uphill anyway.
2. Don't use your bicycle on the road.

Aerobic dance

There is now a big craze for aerobic dance. It offers the promise of

Sports

music, fun, and health.

● Benefits of aerobic dance

1. Improves cardiovascular and muscle fitness. Also will give you some grace of movement.
2. If you are a man, dance classes are a good place to meet women. There are very few men in them, and all the women wear leotards. Even if you don't actually meet them, their presence makes this form of exercise considerably more interesting than jogging.

● Disadvantages of aerobic dance

1. If it includes any real dance exercises, this may demand a flexibility that your body does not have. Attempting to stretch like a dancer can leave you permanently unable to walk.
2. Dancing requires even more coordination than bicycling. These classes can be not only exhausting, but humiliating.

● Dance for the ill

1. Don't go to classes

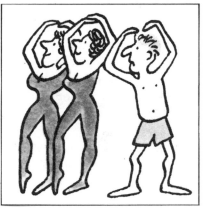
Dance requires coordination.

where the people can touch their toes.
2. Dance only to waltzes.

Sports

The trouble with sports is that in order to become skilled you have to be healthy, or willing to play when you don't feel right. Consequently, although you may play a bit of tennis now and then, you will probably lose most of the time. This makes the sport lose some of its luster.

Don't feel bad. Sports were invented by people with excess energy who wanted to take out all their aggressions on one another. It is not so great to be one of those people. They usually die of heart attacks, no matter how good they are at racqetball. So don't feel pressured to jump into sports. On the other hand, if you have a bit of extra energy sometime, and you want to, then try a sport—take up lawn bowling, take a tennis lesson, try putting.

Stay away from violent sports like squash and volleyball. You don't want to get yourself killed. Some acceptable sports are darts, croquet, friendly golf, and badminton. When you do play, it is probably a good idea to tone the game down by not keeping score. It is not whether you win or lose that counts, but whether you survive the game.

Medication

Human beings, particularly hypochondriacs, cannot live by food and exercise alone. In order to stay alive, they must also take their medicines.

And yet, every time you take a pill you take your life in your hands. Just read the label. It warns you not to take the pills if you have kidney disease. Well, how do you know you don't have kidney disease? Or, it says to stop taking them if you hear a ringing in your ears. The trouble is, you will always hear a ringing in your ears, if you listen.

The end result is that you are in a constant state of fear. All your ailments require medication. And all medications are dangerous. Worse, drugs interact with one another—and with food— unpredictably. Antacids inacti- vate some antibiotics. And there are certain blood pressure drugs which, if combined with avocado, can kill you.*

What is a hypochondriac to do? Is there life without aspirin? Are there colds without antihistamines? Perhaps. But who would want to find out for sure? There is no foolproof way out of this labyrinth of medicinal terror, but you can be informed. You should always have a Merck Manual and a PDR (Physician's Desk Reference, always referred to by its initials) close at hand. This won't stop the drugs from being dangerous, but at least you will know what to be afraid of.

*These are MAO (monoamine oxidase) inhibitors, which interact badly with a chemical called tyramine. There is also tyramine in beer.

How to read a drug label

How to read a drug label

How to read a drug label

Before you delve into the deeper sources of drug information, you have to find out what it is you are taking. The best way to do this is to read the label.

Prescription drugs

Prescription drugs have very uninformative labels; they say things like "iai p smith ac314." Pharmacists seem to strive in their typing for the same level of incomprehensibility that doctors achieve so effortlessly in their handwriting.

So, if your doctor writes you a prescription, don't count on getting anything from the label. Demand an explanation of the drug from him. (*See* The Hippocratic Curse.)

Over-the-counter

Over-the-counter drugs come with a great deal of information. Often they have a tiny pamphlet in the box they come in, as well as a densely printed label. Read everything. The important categories are: *Warning; Drug Interaction Precaution; Usual Dosages;* and *Directions.*

Warning. Read this section first. If it says keep out of the reach of children, you know the medication is dangerous. Don't take it.

Drug Interaction Precaution. Here you will find information such as "Do not take this drug with figs." Or, it may tell you not to take it if you are taking certain kinds of antibiotics, or antidepressants, or blood pressure medication.

It is very likely that you have high blood pressure, an infection, or suffer from depression. It is best to medicate one ailment at a time. Let the others ride. They won't go away, so you'll be able to treat them later.

Usual Dosages. Always take less than they say. You are bound to be more sensitive than a normal person.

Directions. Here the label tells you how to take the pills, and sometimes how often. Frequently it says, "or as directed by a physician." Call your physician. Ask for directions. If he acts unfriendly, say the label told you to get in touch with him.

Drugs

Note: If your label says "Sample. Not for Sale. Research Purposes Only," report your pharmacist to the FBI or the NIH.* But save a few of the pills. They might be a new cure for something you haven't got yet.

Common and dangerous drugs

It was the best of drugs; it was the worst of drugs. For years hypochondriacs have taken aspirin regularly, the way some people wear wolfsbane. Now there has been an aspirin backlash.

True, aspirin is the best pain reliever around. True, it may prevent heart attacks. True, it is the mainstay of drug advertisements. But, it can also make you bleed to death. And it interacts with everything. If you insist on taking aspirin, take the orange-tasting children's kind. You will feel safer. If, however, you think you might be a hemophiliac (Is your blood very liquid?), take something else for your headaches.

Other common drugs can also be dangerous:

Antihistamines. You can't have a cold without antihis-

tamines. And yet, as all hypochondriacs know, the warning on the label says, "May cause drowsiness; therefore, avoid driving a motor vehicle or operating heavy machinery."

If you want to be safe, this means staying away from the food processor. Other machines you should not operate under the influence of antihistamines are lawn mowers (with or without motors), typewriters, televisions, and air conditioners.

Antihistamines may also cause "excitability" according to their labels—not nervousness, or anxiety or restlessness, but excitability. This means that you should never take antihistamines when you are likely to receive good news. Fortunately, you are seldom likely to receive good news.

Valium. These little yellow tablets have become one of the most popular drugs in America. Don't take them unless you can help it. They can become habit-forming. Worse, they can lower sexual desire. Hypochondriacs do not need anything to lower their sexual desire.

Placebos. A placebo is a

*National Institutes of Health.

Drugs

How to take a pill

Once you know what it is you are about to take, and you have momentarily conquered your fears about what the drug will do to you, you have to take the medicine.

Dry pills. These are the pills that are not in capsules. Dry pills taste awful, so the pressure to get them down quickly is intense. Place them far back on the tongue.

Slick pills. These are capsules. You can't taste them unless you chew them, which you should not do. The lack of taste makes them easier to swallow, but they are often huge. Always place them on your tongue so they lie lengthwise from lips to throat.

Water. Always use a big glass of water. Nothing is worse than getting caught short of water with a bad-tasting pill. Pour water into your mouth. Tilt your head back slightly, and swallow. If you lose the pill in your mouth, do not give up and spit everything out into the sink. Just keep drinking water and swallowing until there is no bad taste in your mouth. Then, even if the pill dissolved, you have still managed to swallow most of it.

medically inactive substance given to a patient who is told that it is penicillin, Valium, or some other medication. Doctors sometimes give placebos to patients when they think their complaints are not real. As a hypochondriac you may well be getting placebos.

If so, beware. There is a well-known "placebo effect." Some ailments, completely unimaginary, will respond to placebos just the way they would to the real drugs. The danger lies in the reverse placebo effect. If you are well informed about the side effects of your medication, you may suffer them even if your pill is a placebo.

Drug interactions

Combining drugs can be exceedingly dangerous, the classic case being barbiturates and alcohol. Other dangerous interactions are less well known.

1. Valium and camomile tea. Two powerful tranquilizers. Taking them in combination makes you what Californians call "mellow." Another word for this state of mind is "catatonic." If you find yourself developing a

Drug interactions

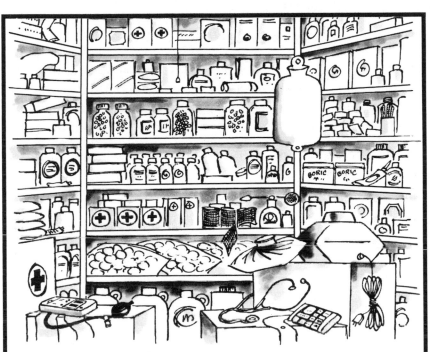

The hypochondriac's medicine cabinet

For headaches:
Aspirin
Tylenol
ice pack

For colds, flu, strep throat, . and pneumonia:
antihistamines
antibiotics
  (penicillin,
  Achromycin,
  Aureomycin,
  Ampicillin,
  Chloromycetin,
  Polycillin, Sumycin,
  tetracycline)
hot water bottle
thermometers
humidifier

For the heart:
stethoscope
stopwatch
blood pressure
  machine
pulse monitor
digitoxin

For injuries:
Iodine
Mercurochrome
Merthiolate
antibacterial ointments
Band-Aids
cotton balls
tourniquets
gauze
tape
Ace bandages
ice pack

For the out-of-doors:
sun lotion
benzocaine
bee sting kit
snakebite kit
hypothermia kit
  (warm blankets,
  thermos, and an at-
  tractive friend)

For the stomach:
Maalox
Gelusil
Di-Gel
ginger ale

For unhappiness:
Elavil
Pertofran
Tofranil
ginger ale

For excess happiness:
Librium
Miltown
Valium
Thorazine

For shock and disappointment:
hot water bottle
thermometers
lots of blankets

Drug interactions

rapport with the breeze, you are on your way to an overdose.

2. Antidepressants and parties. Going out to a party when you are taking an antidepressant can be a double whammy. You can get pathologically happy. You might embarrass yourself.

3. Muscle relaxants and coffee. You end up alert and tense with a body that feels like well-cooked pasta. Not only is this uncomfortable, it can cause a split personality. (*See* In the Mind.)

How long before you die?

We all know that smoking increases our chances of lung cancer, and that there are other risk factors for other diseases—such as high blood pressure for heart disease. But this doesn't tell us what we really want to know. How long have we got left?

So-called healthy people may put this question aside. Hypochondriacs think about it all the time. The following easy quiz will tell you when you will die. Answer all the questions yes or no.

YES NO

- ☐ ☐ *1.* Have you ever smoked cigarettes?
- ☐ ☐ *2.* Do you ever drink alcohol?
- ☐ ☐ *3.* Do you have sex more than once a week?
- ☐ ☐ *4.* Have you ever had a cold?
- ☐ ☐ *5.* Has anyone died in your family?
- ☐ ☐ *6.* Do you think you might have high blood pressure?
- ☐ ☐ *7.* Do other people make you angry?
- ☐ ☐ *8.* Do you make other people angry?
- ☐ ☐ *9.* Do you worry a lot?
- ☐ ☐ *10.* Do you work in a chemical factory?
- ☐ ☐ *11.* Are you divorced?
- ☐ ☐ *12.* Are you married?
- ☐ ☐ *13.* Are you single?
- ☐ ☐ *14.* Are you a member of organized crime?
- ☐ ☐ *15.* Do you hate to exercise?
- ☐ ☐ *16.* Do you like food?
- ☐ ☐ *17.* Are you on a diet?

How long before you die

☐ ☐ *18.* Do you ever eat beef?

☐ ☐ *19.* Do you think brown rice is boring?

☐ ☐ *20.* Do you eat sushi?

☐ ☐ *21.* Do you eat mayonnaise?

☐ ☐ *22.* Do you sunbathe?

☐ ☐ *23.* Have you ever traveled?

☐ ☐ *24.* Have you ever used insect spray?

☐ ☐ *25.* Have you ever used oven cleaner?

☐ ☐ *26.* More than once?

☐ ☐ *27.* Have you ever gone to a movie in a Times Square theater?

☐ ☐ *28.* More than once?

☐ ☐ *29.* Do you take any medications?

☐ ☐ *30.* Are you under the care of a physician?

To score the test, first count up the number of your yes answers. Give yourself four points for every yes answer. Divide the total number of points by 2. Then subtract the result from 70. This is as old as you will ever get.

Example: Ten yes answers (a health fanatic) times 4 is 40. Divide by 2 and you get 20. Subtract from 70 and you get 50.

If you find by doing the quiz that you died several years ago, see your physician immediately.

If you answered yes to questions 10, 14, or 21, there is no need to do the mathematics. You probably won't make it through the next year.

If you answered no to everything, you have a very long, very strange life ahead of you.